THIS BOOK BELONGS TO:

CONTACT INFORMATION	
NAME:	
ADDRESS:	
PHONE:	

START / END DATES

___ / ___ / ___   TO   ___ / ___ / ___

DEDICATION

This book is dedicated to all dedicated pizza lovers out there who love to eat pizza.

Your are my inspiration for producing books and I'm honored to be a part of keeping your pizza reviews organized.

This journal notebook will help you record your details and experience in reviewing each particular restaurant's pizza.

Thoughtfully put together with these sections to record, Date, Pizzeria, Beverage Pairing, Toppings, Cheese, Sauce, Crust, Crust Rating, Style, Freshness, Notes and Overall Rating.

I hope you enjoy each and every slice of pizza you eat while you document your review!

HOW TO USE THIS BOOK:

The purpose of this book is to keep all of your pizza reviews, experiences and findings all in one place. It will help keep you organized.

This Pizza Review Log will allow you to accurately document all the things you want to remember about your experience eating and reviewing pizza. It's a great way to chart your course through the world of pizza.

Here are examples of the prompts for you to fill in and write about your experience and findings in this book:

1. Date - Write the date of your review.
2. Pizzeria - Record the restaurants name.
3. Beverage Pairing - Write what you had to drink.
4. Toppings - Check which toppings were on your pizza: Cheese, Mushrooms, Onions, Pineapple, Bacon, Tuna, Green Pepper, Sausage, Black Olives, Other, Etc.
5. Cheese - Record whether Greasy, Stingy, Smokey, Stinky, Creamy or Salty.
6. Sauce - Check whether it was Sweet, Savory, Tangy, Spicy, Thin, Chunky.
7. Cheese To Sauce Ratio (CSR) - Use check boxes to record ratio.
8. Crust Taste & Size - Record size: Thin, Medium, Large. And Taste: Buttery, Crispy, Spongy, Bubbly, Chewy, Other.
9. Crust Rating - Rate the crust 1-5.
10. Style - Check what the style was: New York, Chicago or Other.
11. Freshness - Rate the freshness 1-5.
12. Notes/ Comment - Blank lined notes for any other information you want to remember such as a favorite recipe or recipes, favorite best, places, special ingredients, special offer, did you have fun, in town or out of town traveling, favorite restaurants, things you need to know, etc.
13. Overall Quality Rating - Rate 1-10 and would you eat here again.

Pizza Log

DATE	
PIZZERIA	
NEIGHBORHOOD	

TOPPINGS

○ CHEESE	○ MUSHROOMS	○ ONIONS
○ PINEAPPLE	○ BACON	○ TUNA
○ GREEN PEPPER	○ SAUSAGE	○ BLACK OLIVES
○ OTHER		

CHEESE

○ GREASY	○ STINGY
○ SMOKEY	○ STINKY
○ CREAMY	○ SALTY

SAUCE

○ SWEET	○ SAVORY
○ TANGY	○ SPICY
○ THIN	○ CHUNKY

CHEESE TO SAUCE RATIO (CSR)

CHEESE	☐☐☐☐☐☐☐
SAUCE	☐☐☐☐☐☐☐

FRESHNESS

○1 ○2 ○3 ○4 ○5

CRUST SIZE	CRUST	
○ THIN	○ BUTTERY	○ CRISPY
○ MEDIUM	○ SPONGY	○ BUBBLY
○ LARGE	○ CHEWY	○ OTHER

CRUST

○1 ○2 ○3 ○4 ○5

STYLE	○ NY ○ CHICAGO ○ OTHER

COMMENTS

MY RATING	○1 ○2 ○3 ○4 ○5 ○6 ○7 ○8 ○9 ○10	EAT AGAIN?	○ YES ○ NO

Pizza Log

DATE	
PIZZERIA	
NEIGHBORHOOD	

TOPPINGS

- ○ CHEESE
- ○ MUSHROOMS
- ○ ONIONS
- ○ PINEAPPLE
- ○ BACON
- ○ TUNA
- ○ GREEN PEPPER
- ○ SAUSAGE
- ○ BLACK OLIVES
- ○ OTHER

CHEESE

- ○ GREASY
- ○ STINGY
- ○ SMOKEY
- ○ STINKY
- ○ CREAMY
- ○ SALTY

SAUCE

- ○ SWEET
- ○ SAVORY
- ○ TANGY
- ○ SPICY
- ○ THIN
- ○ CHUNKY

CHEESE TO SAUCE RATIO (CSR)

CHEESE	☐ ☐ ☐ ☐ ☐ ☐
SAUCE	☐ ☐ ☐ ☐ ☐ ☐

FRESHNESS

○ 1 ○ 2 ○ 3 ○ 4 ○ 5

CRUST SIZE

- ○ THIN
- ○ MEDIUM
- ○ LARGE

CRUST

- ○ BUTTERY
- ○ CRISPY
- ○ SPONGY
- ○ BUBBLY
- ○ CHEWY
- ○ OTHER

CRUST

○ 1 ○ 2 ○ 3 ○ 4 ○ 5

STYLE	○ NY ○ CHICAGO ○ OTHER

COMMENTS

MY RATING	○ 1 ○ 2 ○ 3 ○ 4 ○ 5 ○ 6 ○ 7 ○ 8 ○ 9 ○ 10	EAT AGAIN?	○ YES ○ NO

Pizza Log

DATE	
PIZZERIA	
NEIGHBORHOOD	

TOPPINGS			CHEESE	
○ CHEESE	○ MUSHROOMS	○ ONIONS	○ GREASY	○ STINGY
○ PINEAPPLE	○ BACON	○ TUNA	○ SMOKEY	○ STINKY
○ GREEN PEPPER	○ SAUSAGE	○ BLACK OLIVES	○ CREAMY	○ SALTY
○ OTHER			**SAUCE**	
			○ SWEET	○ SAVORY
			○ TANGY	○ SPICY
			○ THIN	○ CHUNKY

	CHEESE TO SAUCE RATIO (CSR)	
	CHEESE	☐☐☐☐☐☐
FRESHNESS	SAUCE	☐☐☐☐☐☐
○1 ○2 ○3 ○4 ○5		

CRUST SIZE	CRUST		CRUST	
○ THIN	○ BUTTERY	○ CRISPY	○1 ○2 ○3 ○4 ○5	
○ MEDIUM	○ SPONGY	○ BUBBLY		
○ LARGE	○ CHEWY	○ OTHER	STYLE	○ NY ○ CHICAGO ○ OTHER

COMMENTS

MY RATING	○1 ○2 ○3 ○4 ○5 ○6 ○7 ○8 ○9 ○10	EAT AGAIN?	○ YES ○ NO

Pizza Log

DATE	
PIZZERIA	
NEIGHBORHOOD	

TOPPINGS

○ CHEESE	○ MUSHROOMS	○ ONIONS
○ PINEAPPLE	○ BACON	○ TUNA
○ GREEN PEPPER	○ SAUSAGE	○ BLACK OLIVES
○ OTHER		

CHEESE

○ GREASY	○ STINGY
○ SMOKEY	○ STINKY
○ CREAMY	○ SALTY

SAUCE

○ SWEET	○ SAVORY
○ TANGY	○ SPICY
○ THIN	○ CHUNKY

CHEESE TO SAUCE RATIO (CSR)

CHEESE	☐ ☐ ☐ ☐ ☐ ☐
SAUCE	☐ ☐ ☐ ☐ ☐ ☐

FRESHNESS

○ 1   ○ 2   ○ 3   ○ 4   ○ 5

CRUST SIZE

○ THIN
○ MEDIUM
○ LARGE

CRUST

○ BUTTERY	○ CRISPY
○ SPONGY	○ BUBBLY
○ CHEWY	○ OTHER

CRUST

○ 1   ○ 2   ○ 3   ○ 4   ○ 5

STYLE: ○ NY   ○ CHICAGO   ○ OTHER

COMMENTS

MY RATING: ○ 1 ○ 2 ○ 3 ○ 4 ○ 5 ○ 6 ○ 7 ○ 8 ○ 9 ○ 10

EAT AGAIN?: ○ YES   ○ NO

Pizza Log

DATE	
PIZZERIA	
NEIGHBORHOOD	

TOPPINGS			CHEESE	
○ CHEESE	○ MUSHROOMS	○ ONIONS	○ GREASY	○ STINGY
○ PINEAPPLE	○ BACON	○ TUNA	○ SMOKEY	○ STINKY
○ GREEN PEPPER	○ SAUSAGE	○ BLACK OLIVES	○ CREAMY	○ SALTY
○ OTHER			SAUCE	
			○ SWEET	○ SAVORY
			○ TANGY	○ SPICY
			○ THIN	○ CHUNKY
			CHEESE TO SAUCE RATIO (CSR)	
FRESHNESS			CHEESE	☐☐☐☐☐☐
○1 ○2 ○3 ○4 ○5			SAUCE	☐☐☐☐☐☐

CRUST SIZE	CRUST		CRUST	
○ THIN	○ BUTTERY	○ CRISPY	○1 ○2 ○3 ○4 ○5	
○ MEDIUM	○ SPONGY	○ BUBBLY	STYLE	○ NY ○ CHICAGO ○ OTHER
○ LARGE	○ CHEWY	○ OTHER		

COMMENTS

MY RATING	○1 ○2 ○3 ○4 ○5 ○6 ○7 ○8 ○9 ○10	EAT AGAIN?	○ YES ○ NO

Pizza Log

DATE	
PIZZERIA	
NEIGHBORHOOD	

TOPPINGS

○ CHEESE	○ MUSHROOMS	○ ONIONS
○ PINEAPPLE	○ BACON	○ TUNA
○ GREEN PEPPER	○ SAUSAGE	○ BLACK OLIVES
○ OTHER		

CHEESE

○ GREASY	○ STINGY
○ SMOKEY	○ STINKY
○ CREAMY	○ SALTY

SAUCE

○ SWEET	○ SAVORY
○ TANGY	○ SPICY
○ THIN	○ CHUNKY

CHEESE TO SAUCE RATIO (CSR)

CHEESE	☐ ☐ ☐ ☐ ☐ ☐
SAUCE	☐ ☐ ☐ ☐ ☐ ☐

FRESHNESS

○1 ○2 ○3 ○4 ○5

CRUST

CRUST SIZE	CRUST	
○ THIN	○ BUTTERY	○ CRISPY
○ MEDIUM	○ SPONGY	○ BUBBLY
○ LARGE	○ CHEWY	○ OTHER

CRUST

○1 ○2 ○3 ○4 ○5

STYLE	○ NY ○ CHICAGO ○ OTHER

COMMENTS

MY RATING	○1 ○2 ○3 ○4 ○5 ○6 ○7 ○8 ○9 ○10	EAT AGAIN?	○ YES ○ NO

Pizza Log

DATE	
PIZZERIA	
NEIGHBORHOOD	

TOPPINGS

○ CHEESE	○ MUSHROOMS	○ ONIONS
○ PINEAPPLE	○ BACON	○ TUNA
○ GREEN PEPPER	○ SAUSAGE	○ BLACK OLIVES
○ OTHER		

CHEESE

○ GREASY	○ STINGY
○ SMOKEY	○ STINKY
○ CREAMY	○ SALTY

SAUCE

○ SWEET	○ SAVORY
○ TANGY	○ SPICY
○ THIN	○ CHUNKY

CHEESE TO SAUCE RATIO (CSR)

CHEESE	☐ ☐ ☐ ☐ ☐ ☐
SAUCE	☐ ☐ ☐ ☐ ☐ ☐

FRESHNESS

○1 ○2 ○3 ○4 ○5

CRUST SIZE

- ○ THIN
- ○ MEDIUM
- ○ LARGE

CRUST

○ BUTTERY	○ CRISPY
○ SPONGY	○ BUBBLY
○ CHEWY	○ OTHER

CRUST

○1 ○2 ○3 ○4 ○5

STYLE	○ NY ○ CHICAGO ○ OTHER

COMMENTS

MY RATING	○1 ○2 ○3 ○4 ○5 ○6 ○7 ○8 ○9 ○10	EAT AGAIN?	○ YES ○ NO

Pizza Log

DATE	
PIZZERIA	
NEIGHBORHOOD	

TOPPINGS

○ CHEESE	○ MUSHROOMS	○ ONIONS
○ PINEAPPLE	○ BACON	○ TUNA
○ GREEN PEPPER	○ SAUSAGE	○ BLACK OLIVES
○ OTHER		

CHEESE

○ GREASY	○ STINGY
○ SMOKEY	○ STINKY
○ CREAMY	○ SALTY

SAUCE

○ SWEET	○ SAVORY
○ TANGY	○ SPICY
○ THIN	○ CHUNKY

CHEESE TO SAUCE RATIO (CSR)

CHEESE	☐☐☐☐☐☐
SAUCE	☐☐☐☐☐☐

FRESHNESS

○1 ○2 ○3 ○4 ○5

CRUST SIZE / CRUST

CRUST SIZE	CRUST	
○ THIN	○ BUTTERY	○ CRISPY
○ MEDIUM	○ SPONGY	○ BUBBLY
○ LARGE	○ CHEWY	○ OTHER

CRUST

○1 ○2 ○3 ○4 ○5

STYLE	○ NY ○ CHICAGO ○ OTHER

COMMENTS

MY RATING	○1 ○2 ○3 ○4 ○5 ○6 ○7 ○8 ○9 ○10
EAT AGAIN?	○ YES ○ NO

Pizza Log

DATE	
PIZZERIA	
NEIGHBORHOOD	

TOPPINGS

○ CHEESE	○ MUSHROOMS	○ ONIONS
○ PINEAPPLE	○ BACON	○ TUNA
○ GREEN PEPPER	○ SAUSAGE	○ BLACK OLIVES
○ OTHER		

CHEESE

○ GREASY	○ STINGY
○ SMOKEY	○ STINKY
○ CREAMY	○ SALTY

SAUCE

○ SWEET	○ SAVORY
○ TANGY	○ SPICY
○ THIN	○ CHUNKY

CHEESE TO SAUCE RATIO (CSR)

CHEESE	☐ ☐ ☐ ☐ ☐ ☐ ☐
SAUCE	☐ ☐ ☐ ☐ ☐ ☐ ☐

FRESHNESS

○1 ○2 ○3 ○4 ○5

CRUST SIZE	CRUST	
○ THIN	○ BUTTERY	○ CRISPY
○ MEDIUM	○ SPONGY	○ BUBBLY
○ LARGE	○ CHEWY	○ OTHER

CRUST

○1 ○2 ○3 ○4 ○5

STYLE	○ NY ○ CHICAGO ○ OTHER

COMMENTS

MY RATING	○1 ○2 ○3 ○4 ○5 ○6 ○7 ○8 ○9 ○10	EAT AGAIN?	○ YES ○ NO

Pizza Log

DATE	
PIZZERIA	
NEIGHBORHOOD	

TOPPINGS

- ○ CHEESE
- ○ MUSHROOMS
- ○ ONIONS
- ○ PINEAPPLE
- ○ BACON
- ○ TUNA
- ○ GREEN PEPPER
- ○ SAUSAGE
- ○ BLACK OLIVES
- ○ OTHER

CHEESE

- ○ GREASY
- ○ STINGY
- ○ SMOKEY
- ○ STINKY
- ○ CREAMY
- ○ SALTY

SAUCE

- ○ SWEET
- ○ SAVORY
- ○ TANGY
- ○ SPICY
- ○ THIN
- ○ CHUNKY

CHEESE TO SAUCE RATIO (CSR)

CHEESE	☐☐☐☐☐☐
SAUCE	☐☐☐☐☐☐

FRESHNESS

○ 1 ○ 2 ○ 3 ○ 4 ○ 5

CRUST SIZE

- ○ THIN
- ○ MEDIUM
- ○ LARGE

CRUST

- ○ BUTTERY
- ○ CRISPY
- ○ SPONGY
- ○ BUBBLY
- ○ CHEWY
- ○ OTHER

CRUST

○ 1 ○ 2 ○ 3 ○ 4 ○ 5

STYLE: ○ NY ○ CHICAGO ○ OTHER

COMMENTS

MY RATING: ○ 1 ○ 2 ○ 3 ○ 4 ○ 5 ○ 6 ○ 7 ○ 8 ○ 9 ○ 10

EAT AGAIN?: ○ YES ○ NO

Pizza Log

DATE	
PIZZERIA	
NEIGHBORHOOD	

TOPPINGS

○ CHEESE	○ MUSHROOMS	○ ONIONS
○ PINEAPPLE	○ BACON	○ TUNA
○ GREEN PEPPER	○ SAUSAGE	○ BLACK OLIVES
○ OTHER		

CHEESE

○ GREASY	○ STINGY
○ SMOKEY	○ STINKY
○ CREAMY	○ SALTY

SAUCE

○ SWEET	○ SAVORY
○ TANGY	○ SPICY
○ THIN	○ CHUNKY

CHEESE TO SAUCE RATIO (CSR)

CHEESE	☐☐☐☐☐☐
SAUCE	☐☐☐☐☐☐

FRESHNESS

○1 ○2 ○3 ○4 ○5

CRUST

CRUST SIZE	CRUST	
○ THIN	○ BUTTERY	○ CRISPY
○ MEDIUM	○ SPONGY	○ BUBBLY
○ LARGE	○ CHEWY	○ OTHER

CRUST

○1 ○2 ○3 ○4 ○5

STYLE	○ NY ○ CHICAGO ○ OTHER

COMMENTS

MY RATING	○1 ○2 ○3 ○4 ○5 ○6 ○7 ○8 ○9 ○10	EAT AGAIN?	○ YES ○ NO

Pizza Log

DATE	
PIZZERIA	
NEIGHBORHOOD	

TOPPINGS

○ CHEESE	○ MUSHROOMS	○ ONIONS
○ PINEAPPLE	○ BACON	○ TUNA
○ GREEN PEPPER	○ SAUSAGE	○ BLACK OLIVES
○ OTHER		

CHEESE

○ GREASY	○ STINGY
○ SMOKEY	○ STINKY
○ CREAMY	○ SALTY

SAUCE

○ SWEET	○ SAVORY
○ TANGY	○ SPICY
○ THIN	○ CHUNKY

CHEESE TO SAUCE RATIO (CSR)

CHEESE	☐☐☐☐☐☐
SAUCE	☐☐☐☐☐☐

FRESHNESS

○1 ○2 ○3 ○4 ○5

CRUST

CRUST SIZE	CRUST	
○ THIN	○ BUTTERY	○ CRISPY
○ MEDIUM	○ SPONGY	○ BUBBLY
○ LARGE	○ CHEWY	○ OTHER

CRUST

○1 ○2 ○3 ○4 ○5

STYLE	○ NY ○ CHICAGO ○ OTHER

COMMENTS

MY RATING	○1 ○2 ○3 ○4 ○5 ○6 ○7 ○8 ○9 ○10	EAT AGAIN?	○ YES ○ NO

Pizza Log

DATE	
PIZZERIA	
NEIGHBORHOOD	

TOPPINGS			CHEESE	
○ CHEESE	○ MUSHROOMS	○ ONIONS	○ GREASY	○ STINGY
○ PINEAPPLE	○ BACON	○ TUNA	○ SMOKEY	○ STINKY
○ GREEN PEPPER	○ SAUSAGE	○ BLACK OLIVES	○ CREAMY	○ SALTY

○ OTHER

SAUCE	
○ SWEET	○ SAVORY
○ TANGY	○ SPICY
○ THIN	○ CHUNKY

CHEESE TO SAUCE RATIO (CSR)

FRESHNESS		CHEESE	☐☐☐☐☐☐☐
○1 ○2 ○3 ○4 ○5		SAUCE	☐☐☐☐☐☐☐

CRUST SIZE	CRUST		CRUST	
○ THIN	○ BUTTERY	○ CRISPY	○1 ○2 ○3 ○4 ○5	
○ MEDIUM	○ SPONGY	○ BUBBLY	STYLE	○ NY ○ CHICAGO ○ OTHER
○ LARGE	○ CHEWY	○ OTHER		

COMMENTS

MY RATING	○1 ○2 ○3 ○4 ○5 ○6 ○7 ○8 ○9 ○10	EAT AGAIN?	○ YES ○ NO

Pizza Log

DATE	
PIZZERIA	
NEIGHBORHOOD	

TOPPINGS

○ CHEESE	○ MUSHROOMS	○ ONIONS
○ PINEAPPLE	○ BACON	○ TUNA
○ GREEN PEPPER	○ SAUSAGE	○ BLACK OLIVES
○ OTHER		

CHEESE

○ GREASY	○ STINGY
○ SMOKEY	○ STINKY
○ CREAMY	○ SALTY

SAUCE

○ SWEET	○ SAVORY
○ TANGY	○ SPICY
○ THIN	○ CHUNKY

CHEESE TO SAUCE RATIO (CSR)

CHEESE	☐ ☐ ☐ ☐ ☐ ☐
SAUCE	☐ ☐ ☐ ☐ ☐ ☐

FRESHNESS

○ 1   ○ 2   ○ 3   ○ 4   ○ 5

CRUST

CRUST SIZE	CRUST	
○ THIN	○ BUTTERY	○ CRISPY
○ MEDIUM	○ SPONGY	○ BUBBLY
○ LARGE	○ CHEWY	○ OTHER

CRUST

○ 1   ○ 2   ○ 3   ○ 4   ○ 5

STYLE	○ NY ○ CHICAGO ○ OTHER

COMMENTS

MY RATING	○1 ○2 ○3 ○4 ○5 ○6 ○7 ○8 ○9 ○10	EAT AGAIN?	○ YES ○ NO

Pizza Log

DATE	
PIZZERIA	
NEIGHBORHOOD	

TOPPINGS			CHEESE	
○ CHEESE	○ MUSHROOMS	○ ONIONS	○ GREASY	○ STINGY
○ PINEAPPLE	○ BACON	○ TUNA	○ SMOKEY	○ STINKY
○ GREEN PEPPER	○ SAUSAGE	○ BLACK OLIVES	○ CREAMY	○ SALTY
○ OTHER			SAUCE	
			○ SWEET	○ SAVORY
			○ TANGY	○ SPICY
			○ THIN	○ CHUNKY
			CHEESE TO SAUCE RATIO (CSR)	
FRESHNESS			CHEESE	☐☐☐☐☐☐
○1 ○2 ○3 ○4 ○5			SAUCE	☐☐☐☐☐☐

CRUST SIZE	CRUST		CRUST	
○ THIN	○ BUTTERY	○ CRISPY	○1 ○2 ○3 ○4 ○5	
○ MEDIUM	○ SPONGY	○ BUBBLY		
○ LARGE	○ CHEWY	○ OTHER	STYLE	○ NY ○ CHICAGO ○ OTHER

COMMENTS

MY RATING	○1 ○2 ○3 ○4 ○5 ○6 ○7 ○8 ○9 ○10	EAT AGAIN?	○ YES ○ NO

Pizza Log

DATE	
PIZZERIA	
NEIGHBORHOOD	

TOPPINGS

○ CHEESE	○ MUSHROOMS	○ ONIONS
○ PINEAPPLE	○ BACON	○ TUNA
○ GREEN PEPPER	○ SAUSAGE	○ BLACK OLIVES
○ OTHER		

CHEESE

○ GREASY	○ STINGY
○ SMOKEY	○ STINKY
○ CREAMY	○ SALTY

SAUCE

○ SWEET	○ SAVORY
○ TANGY	○ SPICY
○ THIN	○ CHUNKY

CHEESE TO SAUCE RATIO (CSR)

CHEESE	☐☐☐☐☐☐
SAUCE	☐☐☐☐☐☐

FRESHNESS

○1 ○2 ○3 ○4 ○5

CRUST SIZE / CRUST

CRUST SIZE	CRUST	
○ THIN	○ BUTTERY	○ CRISPY
○ MEDIUM	○ SPONGY	○ BUBBLY
○ LARGE	○ CHEWY	○ OTHER

CRUST

○1 ○2 ○3 ○4 ○5

STYLE	○ NY ○ CHICAGO ○ OTHER

COMMENTS

MY RATING ○1 ○2 ○3 ○4 ○5 ○6 ○7 ○8 ○9 ○10

EAT AGAIN? ○ YES ○ NO

Pizza Log

DATE	
PIZZERIA	
NEIGHBORHOOD	

TOPPINGS

○ CHEESE	○ MUSHROOMS	○ ONIONS
○ PINEAPPLE	○ BACON	○ TUNA
○ GREEN PEPPER	○ SAUSAGE	○ BLACK OLIVES

○ OTHER

CHEESE

○ GREASY	○ STINGY
○ SMOKEY	○ STINKY
○ CREAMY	○ SALTY

SAUCE

○ SWEET	○ SAVORY
○ TANGY	○ SPICY
○ THIN	○ CHUNKY

CHEESE TO SAUCE RATIO (CSR)

CHEESE	☐ ☐ ☐ ☐ ☐ ☐
SAUCE	☐ ☐ ☐ ☐ ☐ ☐

FRESHNESS

○ 1   ○ 2   ○ 3   ○ 4   ○ 5

CRUST SIZE

○ THIN	
○ MEDIUM	
○ LARGE	

CRUST

○ BUTTERY	○ CRISPY
○ SPONGY	○ BUBBLY
○ CHEWY	○ OTHER

CRUST

○ 1   ○ 2   ○ 3   ○ 4   ○ 5

STYLE	○ NY ○ CHICAGO ○ OTHER

COMMENTS

MY RATING	○ 1 ○ 2 ○ 3 ○ 4 ○ 5 ○ 6 ○ 7 ○ 8 ○ 9 ○ 10	EAT AGAIN?	○ YES ○ NO

Pizza Log

DATE	
PIZZERIA	
NEIGHBORHOOD	

TOPPINGS

○ CHEESE	○ MUSHROOMS	○ ONIONS
○ PINEAPPLE	○ BACON	○ TUNA
○ GREEN PEPPER	○ SAUSAGE	○ BLACK OLIVES
○ OTHER		

CHEESE

○ GREASY	○ STINGY
○ SMOKEY	○ STINKY
○ CREAMY	○ SALTY

SAUCE

○ SWEET	○ SAVORY
○ TANGY	○ SPICY
○ THIN	○ CHUNKY

CHEESE TO SAUCE RATIO (CSR)

CHEESE	☐☐☐☐☐☐
SAUCE	☐☐☐☐☐☐

FRESHNESS

○1 ○2 ○3 ○4 ○5

CRUST SIZE

○ THIN	
○ MEDIUM	
○ LARGE	

CRUST

○ BUTTERY	○ CRISPY
○ SPONGY	○ BUBBLY
○ CHEWY	○ OTHER

CRUST

○1 ○2 ○3 ○4 ○5

STYLE	○ NY ○ CHICAGO ○ OTHER

COMMENTS

MY RATING	○1 ○2 ○3 ○4 ○5 ○6 ○7 ○8 ○9 ○10	EAT AGAIN?	○ YES ○ NO

Pizza Log

DATE	
PIZZERIA	
NEIGHBORHOOD	

TOPPINGS

○ CHEESE	○ MUSHROOMS	○ ONIONS
○ PINEAPPLE	○ BACON	○ TUNA
○ GREEN PEPPER	○ SAUSAGE	○ BLACK OLIVES
○ OTHER		

CHEESE

○ GREASY	○ STINGY
○ SMOKEY	○ STINKY
○ CREAMY	○ SALTY

SAUCE

○ SWEET	○ SAVORY
○ TANGY	○ SPICY
○ THIN	○ CHUNKY

CHEESE TO SAUCE RATIO (CSR)

CHEESE	☐☐☐☐☐☐
SAUCE	☐☐☐☐☐☐

FRESHNESS

○1 ○2 ○3 ○4 ○5

CRUST

CRUST SIZE	CRUST	
○ THIN	○ BUTTERY	○ CRISPY
○ MEDIUM	○ SPONGY	○ BUBBLY
○ LARGE	○ CHEWY	○ OTHER

CRUST

○1 ○2 ○3 ○4 ○5

STYLE	○ NY ○ CHICAGO ○ OTHER

COMMENTS

MY RATING	○1 ○2 ○3 ○4 ○5 ○6 ○7 ○8 ○9 ○10	EAT AGAIN?	○ YES ○ NO

Pizza Log

DATE	
PIZZERIA	
NEIGHBORHOOD	

TOPPINGS

○ CHEESE	○ MUSHROOMS	○ ONIONS
○ PINEAPPLE	○ BACON	○ TUNA
○ GREEN PEPPER	○ SAUSAGE	○ BLACK OLIVES

○ OTHER

CHEESE

○ GREASY	○ STINGY
○ SMOKEY	○ STINKY
○ CREAMY	○ SALTY

SAUCE

○ SWEET	○ SAVORY
○ TANGY	○ SPICY
○ THIN	○ CHUNKY

CHEESE TO SAUCE RATIO (CSR)

CHEESE	☐☐☐☐☐☐
SAUCE	☐☐☐☐☐☐

FRESHNESS

○1 ○2 ○3 ○4 ○5

CRUST

CRUST SIZE	CRUST	
○ THIN	○ BUTTERY	○ CRISPY
○ MEDIUM	○ SPONGY	○ BUBBLY
○ LARGE	○ CHEWY	○ OTHER

CRUST

○1 ○2 ○3 ○4 ○5

STYLE	○ NY ○ CHICAGO ○ OTHER

COMMENTS

MY RATING	○1 ○2 ○3 ○4 ○5 ○6 ○7 ○8 ○9 ○10	EAT AGAIN?	○ YES ○ NO

Pizza Log

DATE	
PIZZERIA	
NEIGHBORHOOD	

TOPPINGS

○ CHEESE	○ MUSHROOMS	○ ONIONS
○ PINEAPPLE	○ BACON	○ TUNA
○ GREEN PEPPER	○ SAUSAGE	○ BLACK OLIVES

○ OTHER

CHEESE

○ GREASY	○ STINGY
○ SMOKEY	○ STINKY
○ CREAMY	○ SALTY

SAUCE

○ SWEET	○ SAVORY
○ TANGY	○ SPICY
○ THIN	○ CHUNKY

CHEESE TO SAUCE RATIO (CSR)

CHEESE	☐☐☐☐☐☐
SAUCE	☐☐☐☐☐☐

FRESHNESS

○1 ○2 ○3 ○4 ○5

CRUST SIZE

○ THIN	
○ MEDIUM	
○ LARGE	

CRUST

○ BUTTERY	○ CRISPY
○ SPONGY	○ BUBBLY
○ CHEWY	○ OTHER

CRUST

○1 ○2 ○3 ○4 ○5

STYLE ○ NY ○ CHICAGO ○ OTHER

COMMENTS

MY RATING ○1 ○2 ○3 ○4 ○5 ○6 ○7 ○8 ○9 ○10

EAT AGAIN? ○ YES ○ NO

Pizza Log

DATE	
PIZZERIA	
NEIGHBORHOOD	

TOPPINGS

○ CHEESE	○ MUSHROOMS	○ ONIONS
○ PINEAPPLE	○ BACON	○ TUNA
○ GREEN PEPPER	○ SAUSAGE	○ BLACK OLIVES
○ OTHER		

CHEESE

○ GREASY	○ STINGY
○ SMOKEY	○ STINKY
○ CREAMY	○ SALTY

SAUCE

○ SWEET	○ SAVORY
○ TANGY	○ SPICY
○ THIN	○ CHUNKY

CHEESE TO SAUCE RATIO (CSR)

CHEESE	☐☐☐☐☐☐
SAUCE	☐☐☐☐☐☐

FRESHNESS

○1 ○2 ○3 ○4 ○5

CRUST SIZE

○ THIN	
○ MEDIUM	
○ LARGE	

CRUST

○ BUTTERY	○ CRISPY
○ SPONGY	○ BUBBLY
○ CHEWY	○ OTHER

CRUST

○1 ○2 ○3 ○4 ○5

STYLE	○ NY ○ CHICAGO ○ OTHER

COMMENTS

MY RATING	○1 ○2 ○3 ○4 ○5 ○6 ○7 ○8 ○9 ○10	EAT AGAIN?	○ YES ○ NO

Pizza Log

DATE	
PIZZERIA	
NEIGHBORHOOD	

TOPPINGS

○ CHEESE	○ MUSHROOMS	○ ONIONS
○ PINEAPPLE	○ BACON	○ TUNA
○ GREEN PEPPER	○ SAUSAGE	○ BLACK OLIVES
○ OTHER		

CHEESE

○ GREASY	○ STINGY
○ SMOKEY	○ STINKY
○ CREAMY	○ SALTY

SAUCE

○ SWEET	○ SAVORY
○ TANGY	○ SPICY
○ THIN	○ CHUNKY

CHEESE TO SAUCE RATIO (CSR)

CHEESE	☐ ☐ ☐ ☐ ☐ ☐
SAUCE	☐ ☐ ☐ ☐ ☐ ☐

FRESHNESS

○ 1 ○ 2 ○ 3 ○ 4 ○ 5

CRUST SIZE	CRUST	
○ THIN	○ BUTTERY	○ CRISPY
○ MEDIUM	○ SPONGY	○ BUBBLY
○ LARGE	○ CHEWY	○ OTHER

CRUST

○ 1 ○ 2 ○ 3 ○ 4 ○ 5

STYLE	○ NY ○ CHICAGO ○ OTHER

COMMENTS

MY RATING	○ 1 ○ 2 ○ 3 ○ 4 ○ 5 ○ 6 ○ 7 ○ 8 ○ 9 ○ 10	EAT AGAIN?	○ YES ○ NO

Pizza Log

DATE	
PIZZERIA	
NEIGHBORHOOD	

TOPPINGS

○ CHEESE	○ MUSHROOMS	○ ONIONS
○ PINEAPPLE	○ BACON	○ TUNA
○ GREEN PEPPER	○ SAUSAGE	○ BLACK OLIVES
○ OTHER		

CHEESE

○ GREASY	○ STINGY
○ SMOKEY	○ STINKY
○ CREAMY	○ SALTY

SAUCE

○ SWEET	○ SAVORY
○ TANGY	○ SPICY
○ THIN	○ CHUNKY

CHEESE TO SAUCE RATIO (CSR)

CHEESE	☐ ☐ ☐ ☐ ☐ ☐
SAUCE	☐ ☐ ☐ ☐ ☐ ☐

FRESHNESS

○ 1 ○ 2 ○ 3 ○ 4 ○ 5

CRUST SIZE / CRUST

CRUST SIZE	CRUST	
○ THIN	○ BUTTERY	○ CRISPY
○ MEDIUM	○ SPONGY	○ BUBBLY
○ LARGE	○ CHEWY	○ OTHER

CRUST

○ 1 ○ 2 ○ 3 ○ 4 ○ 5

STYLE	○ NY ○ CHICAGO ○ OTHER

COMMENTS

MY RATING	○ 1 ○ 2 ○ 3 ○ 4 ○ 5 ○ 6 ○ 7 ○ 8 ○ 9 ○ 10	EAT AGAIN?	○ YES ○ NO

Pizza Log

DATE	
PIZZERIA	
NEIGHBORHOOD	

TOPPINGS

○ CHEESE	○ MUSHROOMS	○ ONIONS
○ PINEAPPLE	○ BACON	○ TUNA
○ GREEN PEPPER	○ SAUSAGE	○ BLACK OLIVES
○ OTHER		

CHEESE

○ GREASY	○ STINGY
○ SMOKEY	○ STINKY
○ CREAMY	○ SALTY

SAUCE

○ SWEET	○ SAVORY
○ TANGY	○ SPICY
○ THIN	○ CHUNKY

CHEESE TO SAUCE RATIO (CSR)

CHEESE	☐ ☐ ☐ ☐ ☐ ☐
SAUCE	☐ ☐ ☐ ☐ ☐ ☐

FRESHNESS

○ 1 ○ 2 ○ 3 ○ 4 ○ 5

CRUST

CRUST SIZE	CRUST	
○ THIN	○ BUTTERY	○ CRISPY
○ MEDIUM	○ SPONGY	○ BUBBLY
○ LARGE	○ CHEWY	○ OTHER

CRUST

○ 1 ○ 2 ○ 3 ○ 4 ○ 5

STYLE	○ NY ○ CHICAGO ○ OTHER

COMMENTS

MY RATING	○ 1 ○ 2 ○ 3 ○ 4 ○ 5 ○ 6 ○ 7 ○ 8 ○ 9 ○ 10	EAT AGAIN?	○ YES ○ NO

Pizza Log

DATE	
PIZZERIA	
NEIGHBORHOOD	

TOPPINGS			CHEESE	
○ CHEESE	○ MUSHROOMS	○ ONIONS	○ GREASY	○ STINGY
○ PINEAPPLE	○ BACON	○ TUNA	○ SMOKEY	○ STINKY
○ GREEN PEPPER	○ SAUSAGE	○ BLACK OLIVES	○ CREAMY	○ SALTY
○ OTHER			SAUCE	
			○ SWEET	○ SAVORY
			○ TANGY	○ SPICY
			○ THIN	○ CHUNKY
			CHEESE TO SAUCE RATIO (CSR)	
FRESHNESS			CHEESE	☐☐☐☐☐☐
○1 ○2 ○3 ○4 ○5			SAUCE	☐☐☐☐☐☐

CRUST SIZE	CRUST		CRUST	
○ THIN	○ BUTTERY	○ CRISPY	○1 ○2 ○3 ○4 ○5	
○ MEDIUM	○ SPONGY	○ BUBBLY	STYLE	○ NY ○ CHICAGO ○ OTHER
○ LARGE	○ CHEWY	○ OTHER		

COMMENTS

MY RATING	○1 ○2 ○3 ○4 ○5 ○6 ○7 ○8 ○9 ○10	EAT AGAIN?	○ YES ○ NO

Pizza Log

DATE	
PIZZERIA	
NEIGHBORHOOD	

TOPPINGS

○ CHEESE	○ MUSHROOMS	○ ONIONS
○ PINEAPPLE	○ BACON	○ TUNA
○ GREEN PEPPER	○ SAUSAGE	○ BLACK OLIVES
○ OTHER		

CHEESE

○ GREASY	○ STINGY
○ SMOKEY	○ STINKY
○ CREAMY	○ SALTY

SAUCE

○ SWEET	○ SAVORY
○ TANGY	○ SPICY
○ THIN	○ CHUNKY

CHEESE TO SAUCE RATIO (CSR)

CHEESE	☐☐☐☐☐☐
SAUCE	☐☐☐☐☐☐

FRESHNESS

○ 1   ○ 2   ○ 3   ○ 4   ○ 5

CRUST SIZE

○ THIN
○ MEDIUM
○ LARGE

CRUST

○ BUTTERY	○ CRISPY
○ SPONGY	○ BUBBLY
○ CHEWY	○ OTHER

CRUST

○ 1   ○ 2   ○ 3   ○ 4   ○ 5

STYLE	○ NY ○ CHICAGO ○ OTHER

COMMENTS

MY RATING	○ 1 ○ 2 ○ 3 ○ 4 ○ 5 ○ 6 ○ 7 ○ 8 ○ 9 ○ 10	EAT AGAIN?	○ YES ○ NO

Pizza Log

DATE	
PIZZERIA	
NEIGHBORHOOD	

TOPPINGS

○ CHEESE	○ MUSHROOMS	○ ONIONS
○ PINEAPPLE	○ BACON	○ TUNA
○ GREEN PEPPER	○ SAUSAGE	○ BLACK OLIVES
○ OTHER		

CHEESE

○ GREASY	○ STINGY
○ SMOKEY	○ STINKY
○ CREAMY	○ SALTY

SAUCE

○ SWEET	○ SAVORY
○ TANGY	○ SPICY
○ THIN	○ CHUNKY

CHEESE TO SAUCE RATIO (CSR)

CHEESE	☐☐☐☐☐☐
SAUCE	☐☐☐☐☐☐

FRESHNESS

○1 ○2 ○3 ○4 ○5

CRUST SIZE / CRUST

CRUST SIZE	CRUST	
○ THIN	○ BUTTERY	○ CRISPY
○ MEDIUM	○ SPONGY	○ BUBBLY
○ LARGE	○ CHEWY	○ OTHER

CRUST

○1 ○2 ○3 ○4 ○5

STYLE	○ NY ○ CHICAGO ○ OTHER

COMMENTS

MY RATING	○1 ○2 ○3 ○4 ○5 ○6 ○7 ○8 ○9 ○10	EAT AGAIN?	○ YES ○ NO

Pizza Log

DATE	
PIZZERIA	
NEIGHBORHOOD	

TOPPINGS

○ CHEESE	○ MUSHROOMS	○ ONIONS
○ PINEAPPLE	○ BACON	○ TUNA
○ GREEN PEPPER	○ SAUSAGE	○ BLACK OLIVES
○ OTHER		

CHEESE

○ GREASY	○ STINGY
○ SMOKEY	○ STINKY
○ CREAMY	○ SALTY

SAUCE

○ SWEET	○ SAVORY
○ TANGY	○ SPICY
○ THIN	○ CHUNKY

CHEESE TO SAUCE RATIO (CSR)

CHEESE	☐☐☐☐☐☐
SAUCE	☐☐☐☐☐☐

FRESHNESS

○1 ○2 ○3 ○4 ○5

CRUST SIZE

○ THIN	
○ MEDIUM	
○ LARGE	

CRUST

○ BUTTERY	○ CRISPY
○ SPONGY	○ BUBBLY
○ CHEWY	○ OTHER

CRUST

○1 ○2 ○3 ○4 ○5

STYLE	○ NY ○ CHICAGO ○ OTHER

COMMENTS

MY RATING	○1 ○2 ○3 ○4 ○5 ○6 ○7 ○8 ○9 ○10	EAT AGAIN?	○ YES ○ NO

Pizza Log

DATE	
PIZZERIA	
NEIGHBORHOOD	

TOPPINGS

○ CHEESE	○ MUSHROOMS	○ ONIONS
○ PINEAPPLE	○ BACON	○ TUNA
○ GREEN PEPPER	○ SAUSAGE	○ BLACK OLIVES
○ OTHER		

CHEESE

○ GREASY	○ STINGY
○ SMOKEY	○ STINKY
○ CREAMY	○ SALTY

SAUCE

○ SWEET	○ SAVORY
○ TANGY	○ SPICY
○ THIN	○ CHUNKY

CHEESE TO SAUCE RATIO (CSR)

CHEESE	☐☐☐☐☐☐
SAUCE	☐☐☐☐☐☐

FRESHNESS

○1 ○2 ○3 ○4 ○5

CRUST SIZE	CRUST		CRUST
○ THIN	○ BUTTERY	○ CRISPY	○1 ○2 ○3 ○4 ○5
○ MEDIUM	○ SPONGY	○ BUBBLY	
○ LARGE	○ CHEWY	○ OTHER	STYLE: ○ NY ○ CHICAGO ○ OTHER

COMMENTS

MY RATING: ○1 ○2 ○3 ○4 ○5 ○6 ○7 ○8 ○9 ○10

EAT AGAIN? ○ YES ○ NO

Pizza Log

DATE	
PIZZERIA	
NEIGHBORHOOD	

TOPPINGS

			CHEESE	
○ CHEESE	○ MUSHROOMS	○ ONIONS	○ GREASY	○ STINGY
○ PINEAPPLE	○ BACON	○ TUNA	○ SMOKEY	○ STINKY
○ GREEN PEPPER	○ SAUSAGE	○ BLACK OLIVES	○ CREAMY	○ SALTY
○ OTHER			SAUCE	
			○ SWEET	○ SAVORY
			○ TANGY	○ SPICY
			○ THIN	○ CHUNKY

CHEESE TO SAUCE RATIO (CSR)

	FRESHNESS		CHEESE	☐☐☐☐☐☐☐
	○1 ○2 ○3 ○4 ○5		SAUCE	☐☐☐☐☐☐☐

CRUST SIZE	CRUST		CRUST	
○ THIN	○ BUTTERY	○ CRISPY	○1 ○2 ○3 ○4 ○5	
○ MEDIUM	○ SPONGY	○ BUBBLY	STYLE	○ NY ○ CHICAGO ○ OTHER
○ LARGE	○ CHEWY	○ OTHER		

COMMENTS

MY RATING	○1 ○2 ○3 ○4 ○5 ○6 ○7 ○8 ○9 ○10	EAT AGAIN?	○ YES ○ NO

Pizza Log

DATE	
PIZZERIA	
NEIGHBORHOOD	

TOPPINGS

○ CHEESE	○ MUSHROOMS	○ ONIONS
○ PINEAPPLE	○ BACON	○ TUNA
○ GREEN PEPPER	○ SAUSAGE	○ BLACK OLIVES
○ OTHER		

CHEESE

○ GREASY	○ STINGY
○ SMOKEY	○ STINKY
○ CREAMY	○ SALTY

SAUCE

○ SWEET	○ SAVORY
○ TANGY	○ SPICY
○ THIN	○ CHUNKY

CHEESE TO SAUCE RATIO (CSR)

CHEESE	☐ ☐ ☐ ☐ ☐ ☐
SAUCE	☐ ☐ ☐ ☐ ☐ ☐

FRESHNESS

○1 ○2 ○3 ○4 ○5

CRUST SIZE / CRUST

CRUST SIZE	CRUST	
○ THIN	○ BUTTERY	○ CRISPY
○ MEDIUM	○ SPONGY	○ BUBBLY
○ LARGE	○ CHEWY	○ OTHER

CRUST

○1 ○2 ○3 ○4 ○5

STYLE	○ NY ○ CHICAGO ○ OTHER

COMMENTS

MY RATING	○1 ○2 ○3 ○4 ○5 ○6 ○7 ○8 ○9 ○10	EAT AGAIN?	○ YES ○ NO

Pizza Log

DATE	
PIZZERIA	
NEIGHBORHOOD	

TOPPINGS

○ CHEESE	○ MUSHROOMS	○ ONIONS
○ PINEAPPLE	○ BACON	○ TUNA
○ GREEN PEPPER	○ SAUSAGE	○ BLACK OLIVES
○ OTHER		

CHEESE

○ GREASY	○ STINGY
○ SMOKEY	○ STINKY
○ CREAMY	○ SALTY

SAUCE

○ SWEET	○ SAVORY
○ TANGY	○ SPICY
○ THIN	○ CHUNKY

CHEESE TO SAUCE RATIO (CSR)

CHEESE	☐☐☐☐☐☐
SAUCE	☐☐☐☐☐☐

FRESHNESS

○1 ○2 ○3 ○4 ○5

CRUST SIZE

○ THIN
○ MEDIUM
○ LARGE

CRUST

○ BUTTERY	○ CRISPY
○ SPONGY	○ BUBBLY
○ CHEWY	○ OTHER

CRUST

○1 ○2 ○3 ○4 ○5

STYLE	○ NY ○ CHICAGO ○ OTHER

COMMENTS

MY RATING	○1 ○2 ○3 ○4 ○5 ○6 ○7 ○8 ○9 ○10	EAT AGAIN?	○ YES ○ NO

Pizza Log

DATE	
PIZZERIA	
NEIGHBORHOOD	

TOPPINGS

○ CHEESE	○ MUSHROOMS	○ ONIONS
○ PINEAPPLE	○ BACON	○ TUNA
○ GREEN PEPPER	○ SAUSAGE	○ BLACK OLIVES
○ OTHER		

CHEESE

○ GREASY	○ STINGY
○ SMOKEY	○ STINKY
○ CREAMY	○ SALTY

SAUCE

○ SWEET	○ SAVORY
○ TANGY	○ SPICY
○ THIN	○ CHUNKY

CHEESE TO SAUCE RATIO (CSR)

CHEESE	☐ ☐ ☐ ☐ ☐ ☐
SAUCE	☐ ☐ ☐ ☐ ☐ ☐

FRESHNESS

○ 1 ○ 2 ○ 3 ○ 4 ○ 5

CRUST SIZE

○ THIN	
○ MEDIUM	
○ LARGE	

CRUST

○ BUTTERY	○ CRISPY
○ SPONGY	○ BUBBLY
○ CHEWY	○ OTHER

CRUST

○ 1 ○ 2 ○ 3 ○ 4 ○ 5

STYLE	○ NY ○ CHICAGO ○ OTHER

COMMENTS

MY RATING	○ 1 ○ 2 ○ 3 ○ 4 ○ 5 ○ 6 ○ 7 ○ 8 ○ 9 ○ 10	EAT AGAIN?	○ YES ○ NO

Pizza Log

DATE	
PIZZERIA	
NEIGHBORHOOD	

TOPPINGS

○ CHEESE	○ MUSHROOMS	○ ONIONS
○ PINEAPPLE	○ BACON	○ TUNA
○ GREEN PEPPER	○ SAUSAGE	○ BLACK OLIVES
○ OTHER		

CHEESE

○ GREASY	○ STINGY
○ SMOKEY	○ STINKY
○ CREAMY	○ SALTY

SAUCE

○ SWEET	○ SAVORY
○ TANGY	○ SPICY
○ THIN	○ CHUNKY

CHEESE TO SAUCE RATIO (CSR)

CHEESE	☐☐☐☐☐☐
SAUCE	☐☐☐☐☐☐

FRESHNESS

○1 ○2 ○3 ○4 ○5

CRUST SIZE

○ THIN	
○ MEDIUM	
○ LARGE	

CRUST

○ BUTTERY	○ CRISPY
○ SPONGY	○ BUBBLY
○ CHEWY	○ OTHER

CRUST

○1 ○2 ○3 ○4 ○5

STYLE	○ NY ○ CHICAGO ○ OTHER

CUMMENTS

MY RATING	○1 ○2 ○3 ○4 ○5 ○6 ○7 ○8 ○9 ○10	EAT AGAIN?	○ YES ○ NO

Pizza Log

DATE	
PIZZERIA	
NEIGHBORHOOD	

TOPPINGS			CHEESE	
○ CHEESE	○ MUSHROOMS	○ ONIONS	○ GREASY	○ STINGY
○ PINEAPPLE	○ BACON	○ TUNA	○ SMOKEY	○ STINKY
○ GREEN PEPPER	○ SAUSAGE	○ BLACK OLIVES	○ CREAMY	○ SALTY
○ OTHER			SAUCE	
			○ SWEET	○ SAVORY
			○ TANGY	○ SPICY
			○ THIN	○ CHUNKY

			CHEESE TO SAUCE RATIO (CSR)	
	FRESHNESS		CHEESE	☐☐☐☐☐☐☐
	○1 ○2 ○3 ○4 ○5		SAUCE	☐☐☐☐☐☐☐

CRUST SIZE	CRUST		CRUST	
○ THIN	○ BUTTERY	○ CRISPY	○1 ○2 ○3 ○4 ○5	
○ MEDIUM	○ SPONGY	○ BUBBLY	STYLE	○ NY ○ CHICAGO ○ OTHER
○ LARGE	○ CHEWY	○ OTHER		

COMMENTS

MY RATING	○1 ○2 ○3 ○4 ○5 ○6 ○7 ○8 ○9 ○10	EAT AGAIN?	○ YES ○ NO

Pizza Log

DATE	
PIZZERIA	
NEIGHBORHOOD	

TOPPINGS

○ CHEESE	○ MUSHROOMS	○ ONIONS
○ PINEAPPLE	○ BACON	○ TUNA
○ GREEN PEPPER	○ SAUSAGE	○ BLACK OLIVES
○ OTHER		

CHEESE

○ GREASY	○ STINGY
○ SMOKEY	○ STINKY
○ CREAMY	○ SALTY

SAUCE

○ SWEET	○ SAVORY
○ TANGY	○ SPICY
○ THIN	○ CHUNKY

CHEESE TO SAUCE RATIO (CSR)

CHEESE	☐ ☐ ☐ ☐ ☐ ☐
SAUCE	☐ ☐ ☐ ☐ ☐ ☐

FRESHNESS

○ 1   ○ 2   ○ 3   ○ 4   ○ 5

CRUST SIZE	CRUST		CRUST
○ THIN	○ BUTTERY	○ CRISPY	○ 1 ○ 2 ○ 3 ○ 4 ○ 5
○ MEDIUM	○ SPONGY	○ BUBBLY	
○ LARGE	○ CHEWY	○ OTHER	STYLE: ○ NY ○ CHICAGO ○ OTHER

COMMENTS

MY RATING	○1 ○2 ○3 ○4 ○5 ○6 ○7 ○8 ○9 ○10	EAT AGAIN?	○ YES ○ NO

Pizza Log

DATE	
PIZZERIA	
NEIGHBORHOOD	

TOPPINGS

○ CHEESE	○ MUSHROOMS	○ ONIONS
○ PINEAPPLE	○ BACON	○ TUNA
○ GREEN PEPPER	○ SAUSAGE	○ BLACK OLIVES
○ OTHER		

CHEESE

○ GREASY	○ STINGY
○ SMOKEY	○ STINKY
○ CREAMY	○ SALTY

SAUCE

○ SWEET	○ SAVORY
○ TANGY	○ SPICY
○ THIN	○ CHUNKY

CHEESE TO SAUCE RATIO (CSR)

CHEESE	☐☐☐☐☐☐☐
SAUCE	☐☐☐☐☐☐☐

FRESHNESS

○1 ○2 ○3 ○4 ○5

CRUST SIZE	CRUST	
○ THIN	○ BUTTERY	○ CRISPY
○ MEDIUM	○ SPONGY	○ BUBBLY
○ LARGE	○ CHEWY	○ OTHER

CRUST

○1 ○2 ○3 ○4 ○5

STYLE	○ NY ○ CHICAGO ○ OTHER

COMMENTS

MY RATING	○1 ○2 ○3 ○4 ○5 ○6 ○7 ○8 ○9 ○10	EAT AGAIN?	○ YES ○ NO

Pizza Log

DATE	
PIZZERIA	
NEIGHBORHOOD	

TOPPINGS

○ CHEESE	○ MUSHROOMS	○ ONIONS
○ PINEAPPLE	○ BACON	○ TUNA
○ GREEN PEPPER	○ SAUSAGE	○ BLACK OLIVES
○ OTHER		

CHEESE

○ GREASY	○ STINGY
○ SMOKEY	○ STINKY
○ CREAMY	○ SALTY

SAUCE

○ SWEET	○ SAVORY
○ TANGY	○ SPICY
○ THIN	○ CHUNKY

CHEESE TO SAUCE RATIO (CSR)

CHEESE	☐☐☐☐☐☐☐
SAUCE	☐☐☐☐☐☐☐

FRESHNESS

○ 1 ○ 2 ○ 3 ○ 4 ○ 5

CRUST SIZE

○ THIN	
○ MEDIUM	
○ LARGE	

CRUST

○ BUTTERY	○ CRISPY
○ SPONGY	○ BUBBLY
○ CHEWY	○ OTHER

CRUST

○ 1 ○ 2 ○ 3 ○ 4 ○ 5

STYLE	○ NY ○ CHICAGO ○ OTHER

COMMENTS

MY RATING	○ 1 ○ 2 ○ 3 ○ 4 ○ 5 ○ 6 ○ 7 ○ 8 ○ 9 ○ 10	EAT AGAIN?	○ YES ○ NO

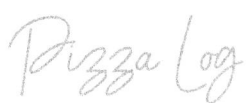

Pizza Log

DATE	
PIZZERIA	
NEIGHBORHOOD	

TOPPINGS			CHEESE	
○ CHEESE	○ MUSHROOMS	○ ONIONS	○ GREASY	○ STINGY
○ PINEAPPLE	○ BACON	○ TUNA	○ SMOKEY	○ STINKY
○ GREEN PEPPER	○ SAUSAGE	○ BLACK OLIVES	○ CREAMY	○ SALTY
○ OTHER			SAUCE	
			○ SWEET	○ SAVORY
			○ TANGY	○ SPICY
			○ THIN	○ CHUNKY
			CHEESE TO SAUCE RATIO (CSR)	
FRESHNESS			CHEESE	☐☐☐☐☐☐☐
○1 ○2 ○3 ○4 ○5			SAUCE	☐☐☐☐☐☐☐

CRUST SIZE	CRUST		CRUST	
○ THIN	○ BUTTERY	○ CRISPY	○1 ○2 ○3 ○4 ○5	
○ MEDIUM	○ SPONGY	○ BUBBLY	STYLE	○ NY ○ CHICAGO ○ OTHER
○ LARGE	○ CHEWY	○ OTHER		

COMMENTS

MY RATING	○1 ○2 ○3 ○4 ○5 ○6 ○7 ○8 ○9 ○10	EAT AGAIN?	○ YES ○ NO

Pizza Log

DATE	
PIZZERIA	
NEIGHBORHOOD	

TOPPINGS

○ CHEESE	○ MUSHROOMS	○ ONIONS
○ PINEAPPLE	○ BACON	○ TUNA
○ GREEN PEPPER	○ SAUSAGE	○ BLACK OLIVES
○ OTHER		

CHEESE

○ GREASY	○ STINGY
○ SMOKEY	○ STINKY
○ CREAMY	○ SALTY

SAUCE

○ SWEET	○ SAVORY
○ TANGY	○ SPICY
○ THIN	○ CHUNKY

CHEESE TO SAUCE RATIO (CSR)

CHEESE	☐☐☐☐☐☐☐
SAUCE	☐☐☐☐☐☐☐

FRESHNESS

○1　○2　○3　○4　○5

CRUST SIZE

○ THIN
○ MEDIUM
○ LARGE

CRUST

○ BUTTERY	○ CRISPY
○ SPONGY	○ BUBBLY
○ CHEWY	○ OTHER

CRUST

○1　○2　○3　○4　○5

STYLE	○ NY　○ CHICAGO　○ OTHER

COMMENTS

MY RATING	○1 ○2 ○3 ○4 ○5 ○6 ○7 ○8 ○9 ○10	EAT AGAIN?	○ YES ○ NO

Pizza Log

DATE	
PIZZERIA	
NEIGHBORHOOD	

TOPPINGS			CHEESE	
○ CHEESE	○ MUSHROOMS	○ ONIONS	○ GREASY	○ STINGY
○ PINEAPPLE	○ BACON	○ TUNA	○ SMOKEY	○ STINKY
○ GREEN PEPPER	○ SAUSAGE	○ BLACK OLIVES	○ CREAMY	○ SALTY
○ OTHER			SAUCE	
			○ SWEET	○ SAVORY
			○ TANGY	○ SPICY
			○ THIN	○ CHUNKY
			CHEESE TO SAUCE RATIO (CSR)	
FRESHNESS			CHEESE	☐☐☐☐☐☐
○1 ○2 ○3 ○4 ○5			SAUCE	☐☐☐☐☐☐

CRUST SIZE	CRUST		CRUST	
○ THIN	○ BUTTERY	○ CRISPY	○1 ○2 ○3 ○4 ○5	
○ MEDIUM	○ SPONGY	○ BUBBLY	STYLE	○ NY ○ CHICAGO ○ OTHER
○ LARGE	○ CHEWY	○ OTHER		

COMMENTS

MY RATING	○1 ○2 ○3 ○4 ○5 ○6 ○7 ○8 ○9 ○10	EAT AGAIN?	○ YES ○ NO

Pizza Log

DATE	
PIZZERIA	
NEIGHBORHOOD	

TOPPINGS			CHEESE	
○ CHEESE	○ MUSHROOMS	○ ONIONS	○ GREASY	○ STINGY
○ PINEAPPLE	○ BACON	○ TUNA	○ SMOKEY	○ STINKY
○ GREEN PEPPER	○ SAUSAGE	○ BLACK OLIVES	○ CREAMY	○ SALTY
○ OTHER			SAUCE	
			○ SWEET	○ SAVORY
			○ TANGY	○ SPICY
			○ THIN	○ CHUNKY

		CHEESE TO SAUCE RATIO (CSR)	
FRESHNESS		CHEESE	☐☐☐☐☐☐
○1 ○2 ○3 ○4 ○5		SAUCE	☐☐☐☐☐☐

CRUST SIZE	CRUST		CRUST	
○ THIN	○ BUTTERY	○ CRISPY	○1 ○2 ○3 ○4 ○5	
○ MEDIUM	○ SPONGY	○ BUBBLY		
○ LARGE	○ CHEWY	○ OTHER	STYLE	○ NY ○ CHICAGO ○ OTHER

COMMENTS

MY RATING	○1 ○2 ○3 ○4 ○5 ○6 ○7 ○8 ○9 ○10	EAT AGAIN?	○ YES ○ NO

Pizza Log

DATE	
PIZZERIA	
NEIGHBORHOOD	

TOPPINGS

○ CHEESE	○ MUSHROOMS	○ ONIONS
○ PINEAPPLE	○ BACON	○ TUNA
○ GREEN PEPPER	○ SAUSAGE	○ BLACK OLIVES
○ OTHER		

CHEESE

○ GREASY	○ STINGY
○ SMOKEY	○ STINKY
○ CREAMY	○ SALTY

SAUCE

○ SWEET	○ SAVORY
○ TANGY	○ SPICY
○ THIN	○ CHUNKY

CHEESE TO SAUCE RATIO (CSR)

CHEESE	☐ ☐ ☐ ☐ ☐ ☐ ☐
SAUCE	☐ ☐ ☐ ☐ ☐ ☐ ☐

FRESHNESS

○1　○2　○3　○4　○5

CRUST SIZE

○ THIN	
○ MEDIUM	
○ LARGE	

CRUST

○ BUTTERY	○ CRISPY
○ SPONGY	○ BUBBLY
○ CHEWY	○ OTHER

CRUST

○1　○2　○3　○4　○5

STYLE	○ NY ○ CHICAGO ○ OTHER

COMMENTS

MY RATING	○1 ○2 ○3 ○4 ○5 ○6 ○7 ○8 ○9 ○10	EAT AGAIN?	○ YES ○ NO

Pizza Log

DATE	
PIZZERIA	
NEIGHBORHOOD	

TOPPINGS			CHEESE	
○ CHEESE	○ MUSHROOMS	○ ONIONS	○ GREASY	○ STINGY
○ PINEAPPLE	○ BACON	○ TUNA	○ SMOKEY	○ STINKY
○ GREEN PEPPER	○ SAUSAGE	○ BLACK OLIVES	○ CREAMY	○ SALTY

OTHER		SAUCE	
○ OTHER		○ SWEET	○ SAVORY
		○ TANGY	○ SPICY
		○ THIN	○ CHUNKY

CHEESE TO SAUCE RATIO (CSR)

FRESHNESS	CHEESE	☐☐☐☐☐☐☐
○1 ○2 ○3 ○4 ○5	SAUCE	☐☐☐☐☐☐☐

CRUST SIZE	CRUST		CRUST
○ THIN	○ BUTTERY	○ CRISPY	○1 ○2 ○3 ○4 ○5
○ MEDIUM	○ SPONGY	○ BUBBLY	
○ LARGE	○ CHEWY	○ OTHER	STYLE: ○ NY ○ CHICAGO ○ OTHER

COMMENTS

MY RATING	○1 ○2 ○3 ○4 ○5 ○6 ○7 ○8 ○9 ○10	EAT AGAIN?	○ YES ○ NO

Pizza Log

DATE	
PIZZERIA	
NEIGHBORHOOD	

TOPPINGS

- ○ CHEESE
- ○ MUSHROOMS
- ○ ONIONS
- ○ PINEAPPLE
- ○ BACON
- ○ TUNA
- ○ GREEN PEPPER
- ○ SAUSAGE
- ○ BLACK OLIVES
- ○ OTHER

CHEESE

- ○ GREASY
- ○ STINGY
- ○ SMOKEY
- ○ STINKY
- ○ CREAMY
- ○ SALTY

SAUCE

- ○ SWEET
- ○ SAVORY
- ○ TANGY
- ○ SPICY
- ○ THIN
- ○ CHUNKY

CHEESE TO SAUCE RATIO (CSR)

CHEESE	☐ ☐ ☐ ☐ ☐ ☐
SAUCE	☐ ☐ ☐ ☐ ☐ ☐

FRESHNESS

○ 1 ○ 2 ○ 3 ○ 4 ○ 5

CRUST SIZE

- ○ THIN
- ○ MEDIUM
- ○ LARGE

CRUST

- ○ BUTTERY
- ○ CRISPY
- ○ SPONGY
- ○ BUBBLY
- ○ CHEWY
- ○ OTHER

CRUST

○ 1 ○ 2 ○ 3 ○ 4 ○ 5

STYLE	○ NY ○ CHICAGO ○ OTHER

COMMENTS

| MY RATING | ○ 1 ○ 2 ○ 3 ○ 4 ○ 5 ○ 6 ○ 7 ○ 8 ○ 9 ○ 10 | EAT AGAIN? | ○ YES ○ NO |

Pizza Log

DATE	
PIZZERIA	
NEIGHBORHOOD	

TOPPINGS

○ CHEESE	○ MUSHROOMS	○ ONIONS
○ PINEAPPLE	○ BACON	○ TUNA
○ GREEN PEPPER	○ SAUSAGE	○ BLACK OLIVES
○ OTHER		

CHEESE

○ GREASY	○ STINGY
○ SMOKEY	○ STINKY
○ CREAMY	○ SALTY

SAUCE

○ SWEET	○ SAVORY
○ TANGY	○ SPICY
○ THIN	○ CHUNKY

CHEESE TO SAUCE RATIO (CSR)

CHEESE	☐☐☐☐☐☐
SAUCE	☐☐☐☐☐☐

FRESHNESS

○1 ○2 ○3 ○4 ○5

CRUST

CRUST SIZE	CRUST	
○ THIN	○ BUTTERY	○ CRISPY
○ MEDIUM	○ SPONGY	○ BUBBLY
○ LARGE	○ CHEWY	○ OTHER

CRUST

○1 ○2 ○3 ○4 ○5

STYLE	○ NY ○ CHICAGO ○ OTHER

COMMENTS

MY RATING	○1 ○2 ○3 ○4 ○5 ○6 ○7 ○8 ○9 ○10	EAT AGAIN?	○ YES ○ NO

Pizza Log

DATE	
PIZZERIA	
NEIGHBORHOOD	

TOPPINGS

○ CHEESE	○ MUSHROOMS	○ ONIONS
○ PINEAPPLE	○ BACON	○ TUNA
○ GREEN PEPPER	○ SAUSAGE	○ BLACK OLIVES
○ OTHER		

CHEESE

○ GREASY	○ STINGY
○ SMOKEY	○ STINKY
○ CREAMY	○ SALTY

SAUCE

○ SWEET	○ SAVORY
○ TANGY	○ SPICY
○ THIN	○ CHUNKY

CHEESE TO SAUCE RATIO (CSR)

CHEESE	☐☐☐☐☐☐
SAUCE	☐☐☐☐☐☐

FRESHNESS

○1 ○2 ○3 ○4 ○5

CRUST SIZE	CRUST	
○ THIN	○ BUTTERY	○ CRISPY
○ MEDIUM	○ SPONGY	○ BUBBLY
○ LARGE	○ CHEWY	○ OTHER

CRUST

○1 ○2 ○3 ○4 ○5

STYLE	○ NY ○ CHICAGO ○ OTHER

COMMENTS

MY RATING	○1 ○2 ○3 ○4 ○5 ○6 ○7 ○8 ○9 ○10	EAT AGAIN?	○ YES ○ NO

Pizza Log

DATE	
PIZZERIA	
NEIGHBORHOOD	

TOPPINGS

○ CHEESE	○ MUSHROOMS	○ ONIONS
○ PINEAPPLE	○ BACON	○ TUNA
○ GREEN PEPPER	○ SAUSAGE	○ BLACK OLIVES
○ OTHER		

CHEESE

○ GREASY	○ STINGY
○ SMOKEY	○ STINKY
○ CREAMY	○ SALTY

SAUCE

○ SWEET	○ SAVORY
○ TANGY	○ SPICY
○ THIN	○ CHUNKY

CHEESE TO SAUCE RATIO (CSR)

CHEESE	☐ ☐ ☐ ☐ ☐ ☐
SAUCE	☐ ☐ ☐ ☐ ☐ ☐

FRESHNESS

○ 1 ○ 2 ○ 3 ○ 4 ○ 5

CRUST SIZE

○ THIN	
○ MEDIUM	
○ LARGE	

CRUST

○ BUTTERY	○ CRISPY
○ SPONGY	○ BUBBLY
○ CHEWY	○ OTHER

CRUST

○ 1 ○ 2 ○ 3 ○ 4 ○ 5

STYLE	○ NY ○ CHICAGO ○ OTHER

COMMENTS

MY RATING	○ 1 ○ 2 ○ 3 ○ 4 ○ 5 ○ 6 ○ 7 ○ 8 ○ 9 ○ 10	EAT AGAIN?	○ YES ○ NO

Pizza Log

DATE	
PIZZERIA	
NEIGHBORHOOD	

TOPPINGS

- ○ CHEESE
- ○ MUSHROOMS
- ○ ONIONS
- ○ PINEAPPLE
- ○ BACON
- ○ TUNA
- ○ GREEN PEPPER
- ○ SAUSAGE
- ○ BLACK OLIVES
- ○ OTHER

CHEESE

- ○ GREASY
- ○ STINGY
- ○ SMOKEY
- ○ STINKY
- ○ CREAMY
- ○ SALTY

SAUCE

- ○ SWEET
- ○ SAVORY
- ○ TANGY
- ○ SPICY
- ○ THIN
- ○ CHUNKY

CHEESE TO SAUCE RATIO (CSR)

CHEESE	☐☐☐☐☐☐
SAUCE	☐☐☐☐☐☐

FRESHNESS

○ 1 ○ 2 ○ 3 ○ 4 ○ 5

CRUST SIZE

- ○ THIN
- ○ MEDIUM
- ○ LARGE

CRUST

- ○ BUTTERY
- ○ CRISPY
- ○ SPONGY
- ○ BUBBLY
- ○ CHEWY
- ○ OTHER

CRUST

○ 1 ○ 2 ○ 3 ○ 4 ○ 5

STYLE: ○ NY ○ CHICAGO ○ OTHER

COMMENTS

MY RATING: ○ 1 ○ 2 ○ 3 ○ 4 ○ 5 ○ 6 ○ 7 ○ 8 ○ 9 ○ 10

EAT AGAIN? ○ YES ○ NO

Pizza Log

DATE	
PIZZERIA	
NEIGHBORHOOD	

TOPPINGS

○ CHEESE	○ MUSHROOMS	○ ONIONS
○ PINEAPPLE	○ BACON	○ TUNA
○ GREEN PEPPER	○ SAUSAGE	○ BLACK OLIVES
○ OTHER		

CHEESE

○ GREASY	○ STINGY
○ SMOKEY	○ STINKY
○ CREAMY	○ SALTY

SAUCE

○ SWEET	○ SAVORY
○ TANGY	○ SPICY
○ THIN	○ CHUNKY

CHEESE TO SAUCE RATIO (CSR)

CHEESE	☐ ☐ ☐ ☐ ☐ ☐
SAUCE	☐ ☐ ☐ ☐ ☐ ☐

FRESHNESS

○ 1   ○ 2   ○ 3   ○ 4   ○ 5

CRUST SIZE

○ THIN	
○ MEDIUM	
○ LARGE	

CRUST

○ BUTTERY	○ CRISPY
○ SPONGY	○ BUBBLY
○ CHEWY	○ OTHER

CRUST

○ 1   ○ 2   ○ 3   ○ 4   ○ 5

STYLE	○ NY ○ CHICAGO ○ OTHER

COMMENTS

MY RATING	○ 1 ○ 2 ○ 3 ○ 4 ○ 5 ○ 6 ○ 7 ○ 8 ○ 9 ○ 10
EAT AGAIN?	○ YES ○ NO

Pizza Log

DATE	
PIZZERIA	
NEIGHBORHOOD	

TOPPINGS

○ CHEESE	○ MUSHROOMS	○ ONIONS
○ PINEAPPLE	○ BACON	○ TUNA
○ GREEN PEPPER	○ SAUSAGE	○ BLACK OLIVES
○ OTHER		

CHEESE

○ GREASY	○ STINGY
○ SMOKEY	○ STINKY
○ CREAMY	○ SALTY

SAUCE

○ SWEET	○ SAVORY
○ TANGY	○ SPICY
○ THIN	○ CHUNKY

CHEESE TO SAUCE RATIO (CSR)

CHEESE	☐ ☐ ☐ ☐ ☐ ☐ ☐
SAUCE	☐ ☐ ☐ ☐ ☐ ☐ ☐

FRESHNESS

○1　○2　○3　○4　○5

CRUST SIZE

○ THIN	
○ MEDIUM	
○ LARGE	

CRUST

○ BUTTERY	○ CRISPY
○ SPONGY	○ BUBBLY
○ CHEWY	○ OTHER

CRUST

○1　○2　○3　○4　○5

STYLE	○ NY　○ CHICAGO　○ OTHER

COMMENTS

MY RATING	○1 ○2 ○3 ○4 ○5 ○6 ○7 ○8 ○9 ○10
EAT AGAIN?	○ YES ○ NO

Pizza Log

DATE	
PIZZERIA	
NEIGHBORHOOD	

TOPPINGS

○ CHEESE	○ MUSHROOMS	○ ONIONS
○ PINEAPPLE	○ BACON	○ TUNA
○ GREEN PEPPER	○ SAUSAGE	○ BLACK OLIVES

○ OTHER

CHEESE

○ GREASY	○ STINGY
○ SMOKEY	○ STINKY
○ CREAMY	○ SALTY

SAUCE

○ SWEET	○ SAVORY
○ TANGY	○ SPICY
○ THIN	○ CHUNKY

CHEESE TO SAUCE RATIO (CSR)

CHEESE	☐ ☐ ☐ ☐ ☐ ☐
SAUCE	☐ ☐ ☐ ☐ ☐ ☐

FRESHNESS

○1 ○2 ○3 ○4 ○5

CRUST SIZE

	CRUST		CRUST
○ THIN	○ BUTTERY	○ CRISPY	○1 ○2 ○3 ○4 ○5
○ MEDIUM	○ SPONGY	○ BUBBLY	
○ LARGE	○ CHEWY	○ OTHER	STYLE: ○ NY ○ CHICAGO ○ OTHER

COMMENTS

MY RATING	○1 ○2 ○3 ○4 ○5 ○6 ○7 ○8 ○9 ○10	EAT AGAIN?	○ YES ○ NO

Pizza Log

DATE	
PIZZERIA	
NEIGHBORHOOD	

TOPPINGS

○ CHEESE	○ MUSHROOMS	○ ONIONS
○ PINEAPPLE	○ BACON	○ TUNA
○ GREEN PEPPER	○ SAUSAGE	○ BLACK OLIVES
○ OTHER		

CHEESE

○ GREASY	○ STINGY
○ SMOKEY	○ STINKY
○ CREAMY	○ SALTY

SAUCE

○ SWEET	○ SAVORY
○ TANGY	○ SPICY
○ THIN	○ CHUNKY

CHEESE TO SAUCE RATIO (CSR)

CHEESE	☐ ☐ ☐ ☐ ☐ ☐
SAUCE	☐ ☐ ☐ ☐ ☐ ☐

FRESHNESS

○ 1 ○ 2 ○ 3 ○ 4 ○ 5

CRUST SIZE / CRUST

CRUST SIZE	CRUST	
○ THIN	○ BUTTERY	○ CRISPY
○ MEDIUM	○ SPONGY	○ BUBBLY
○ LARGE	○ CHEWY	○ OTHER

CRUST

○ 1 ○ 2 ○ 3 ○ 4 ○ 5

STYLE	○ NY ○ CHICAGO ○ OTHER

COMMENTS

MY RATING	○ 1 ○ 2 ○ 3 ○ 4 ○ 5 ○ 6 ○ 7 ○ 8 ○ 9 ○ 10	EAT AGAIN?	○ YES ○ NO

Pizza Log

DATE	
PIZZERIA	
NEIGHBORHOOD	

TOPPINGS

○ CHEESE	○ MUSHROOMS	○ ONIONS
○ PINEAPPLE	○ BACON	○ TUNA
○ GREEN PEPPER	○ SAUSAGE	○ BLACK OLIVES
○ OTHER		

CHEESE

○ GREASY	○ STINGY
○ SMOKEY	○ STINKY
○ CREAMY	○ SALTY

SAUCE

○ SWEET	○ SAVORY
○ TANGY	○ SPICY
○ THIN	○ CHUNKY

CHEESE TO SAUCE RATIO (CSR)

CHEESE	☐☐☐☐☐☐
SAUCE	☐☐☐☐☐☐

FRESHNESS

○ 1 ○ 2 ○ 3 ○ 4 ○ 5

CRUST SIZE

○ THIN	
○ MEDIUM	
○ LARGE	

CRUST

○ BUTTERY	○ CRISPY
○ SPONGY	○ BUBBLY
○ CHEWY	○ OTHER

CRUST

○ 1 ○ 2 ○ 3 ○ 4 ○ 5

STYLE	○ NY ○ CHICAGO ○ OTHER

COMMENTS

MY RATING	○ 1 ○ 2 ○ 3 ○ 4 ○ 5 ○ 6 ○ 7 ○ 8 ○ 9 ○ 10	EAT AGAIN?	○ YES ○ NO

Pizza Log

DATE	
PIZZERIA	
NEIGHBORHOOD	

TOPPINGS

○ CHEESE	○ MUSHROOMS	○ ONIONS
○ PINEAPPLE	○ BACON	○ TUNA
○ GREEN PEPPER	○ SAUSAGE	○ BLACK OLIVES
○ OTHER		

CHEESE

○ GREASY	○ STINGY
○ SMOKEY	○ STINKY
○ CREAMY	○ SALTY

SAUCE

○ SWEET	○ SAVORY
○ TANGY	○ SPICY
○ THIN	○ CHUNKY

CHEESE TO SAUCE RATIO (CSR)

CHEESE	☐☐☐☐☐☐
SAUCE	☐☐☐☐☐☐

FRESHNESS

○1 ○2 ○3 ○4 ○5

CRUST

CRUST SIZE	CRUST	
○ THIN	○ BUTTERY	○ CRISPY
○ MEDIUM	○ SPONGY	○ BUBBLY
○ LARGE	○ CHEWY	○ OTHER

CRUST

○1 ○2 ○3 ○4 ○5

STYLE	○ NY ○ CHICAGO ○ OTHER

COMMENTS

MY RATING	○1 ○2 ○3 ○4 ○5 ○6 ○7 ○8 ○9 ○10	EAT AGAIN?	○ YES ○ NO

Pizza Log

DATE	
PIZZERIA	
NEIGHBORHOOD	

TOPPINGS

○ CHEESE	○ MUSHROOMS	○ ONIONS
○ PINEAPPLE	○ BACON	○ TUNA
○ GREEN PEPPER	○ SAUSAGE	○ BLACK OLIVES
○ OTHER		

CHEESE

○ GREASY	○ STINGY
○ SMOKEY	○ STINKY
○ CREAMY	○ SALTY

SAUCE

○ SWEET	○ SAVORY
○ TANGY	○ SPICY
○ THIN	○ CHUNKY

CHEESE TO SAUCE RATIO (CSR)

CHEESE	☐☐☐☐☐☐☐
SAUCE	☐☐☐☐☐☐☐

FRESHNESS

○1 ○2 ○3 ○4 ○5

CRUST SIZE

○ THIN
○ MEDIUM
○ LARGE

CRUST

○ BUTTERY	○ CRISPY
○ SPONGY	○ BUBBLY
○ CHEWY	○ OTHER

CRUST

○1 ○2 ○3 ○4 ○5

STYLE	○ NY ○ CHICAGO ○ OTHER

COMMENTS

MY RATING	○1 ○2 ○3 ○4 ○5 ○6 ○7 ○8 ○9 ○10	EAT AGAIN?	○ YES ○ NO

Pizza Log

DATE	
PIZZERIA	
NEIGHBORHOOD	

TOPPINGS

○ CHEESE	○ MUSHROOMS	○ ONIONS
○ PINEAPPLE	○ BACON	○ TUNA
○ GREEN PEPPER	○ SAUSAGE	○ BLACK OLIVES
○ OTHER		

CHEESE

○ GREASY	○ STINGY
○ SMOKEY	○ STINKY
○ CREAMY	○ SALTY

SAUCE

○ SWEET	○ SAVORY
○ TANGY	○ SPICY
○ THIN	○ CHUNKY

CHEESE TO SAUCE RATIO (CSR)

CHEESE	☐ ☐ ☐ ☐ ☐ ☐
SAUCE	☐ ☐ ☐ ☐ ☐ ☐

FRESHNESS

○1 ○2 ○3 ○4 ○5

CRUST SIZE / CRUST

CRUST SIZE	CRUST	
○ THIN	○ BUTTERY	○ CRISPY
○ MEDIUM	○ SPONGY	○ BUBBLY
○ LARGE	○ CHEWY	○ OTHER

CRUST

○1 ○2 ○3 ○4 ○5

STYLE	○ NY ○ CHICAGO ○ OTHER

COMMENTS

MY RATING	○1 ○2 ○3 ○4 ○5 ○6 ○7 ○8 ○9 ○10	EAT AGAIN?	○ YES ○ NO

Pizza Log

DATE	
PIZZERIA	
NEIGHBORHOOD	

TOPPINGS			CHEESE	
○ CHEESE	○ MUSHROOMS	○ ONIONS	○ GREASY	○ STINGY
○ PINEAPPLE	○ BACON	○ TUNA	○ SMOKEY	○ STINKY
○ GREEN PEPPER	○ SAUSAGE	○ BLACK OLIVES	○ CREAMY	○ SALTY
○ OTHER			SAUCE	
			○ SWEET	○ SAVORY
			○ TANGY	○ SPICY
			○ THIN	○ CHUNKY
			CHEESE TO SAUCE RATIO (CSR)	
FRESHNESS			CHEESE	☐☐☐☐☐☐
	○1 ○2 ○3 ○4 ○5		SAUCE	☐☐☐☐☐☐

CRUST SIZE	CRUST		CRUST	
○ THIN	○ BUTTERY	○ CRISPY	○1 ○2 ○3 ○4 ○5	
○ MEDIUM	○ SPONGY	○ BUBBLY		
○ LARGE	○ CHEWY	○ OTHER	STYLE	○ NY ○ CHICAGO ○ OTHER

COMMENTS

MY RATING	○1 ○2 ○3 ○4 ○5 ○6 ○7 ○8 ○9 ○10	EAT AGAIN?	○ YES ○ NO

Pizza Log

DATE	
PIZZERIA	
NEIGHBORHOOD	

TOPPINGS

○ CHEESE	○ MUSHROOMS	○ ONIONS
○ PINEAPPLE	○ BACON	○ TUNA
○ GREEN PEPPER	○ SAUSAGE	○ BLACK OLIVES

○ OTHER

CHEESE

○ GREASY	○ STINGY
○ SMOKEY	○ STINKY
○ CREAMY	○ SALTY

SAUCE

○ SWEET	○ SAVORY
○ TANGY	○ SPICY
○ THIN	○ CHUNKY

CHEESE TO SAUCE RATIO (CSR)

CHEESE	☐☐☐☐☐☐
SAUCE	☐☐☐☐☐☐

FRESHNESS

○1 ○2 ○3 ○4 ○5

CRUST SIZE	CRUST	
○ THIN	○ BUTTERY	○ CRISPY
○ MEDIUM	○ SPONGY	○ BUBBLY
○ LARGE	○ CHEWY	○ OTHER

CRUST

○1 ○2 ○3 ○4 ○5

STYLE	○ NY ○ CHICAGO ○ OTHER

COMMENTS

MY RATING	○1 ○2 ○3 ○4 ○5 ○6 ○7 ○8 ○9 ○10	EAT AGAIN?	○ YES ○ NO

Pizza Log

DATE	
PIZZERIA	
NEIGHBORHOOD	

TOPPINGS

○ CHEESE	○ MUSHROOMS	○ ONIONS
○ PINEAPPLE	○ BACON	○ TUNA
○ GREEN PEPPER	○ SAUSAGE	○ BLACK OLIVES

○ OTHER

CHEESE

○ GREASY	○ STINGY
○ SMOKEY	○ STINKY
○ CREAMY	○ SALTY

SAUCE

○ SWEET	○ SAVORY
○ TANGY	○ SPICY
○ THIN	○ CHUNKY

CHEESE TO SAUCE RATIO (CSR)

CHEESE	☐ ☐ ☐ ☐ ☐ ☐ ☐
SAUCE	☐ ☐ ☐ ☐ ☐ ☐ ☐

FRESHNESS

○1 ○2 ○3 ○4 ○5

CRUST SIZE	CRUST	
○ THIN	○ BUTTERY	○ CRISPY
○ MEDIUM	○ SPONGY	○ BUBBLY
○ LARGE	○ CHEWY	○ OTHER

CRUST

○1 ○2 ○3 ○4 ○5

STYLE	○ NY ○ CHICAGO ○ OTHER

COMMENTS

MY RATING	○1 ○2 ○3 ○4 ○5 ○6 ○7 ○8 ○9 ○10	EAT AGAIN?	○ YES ○ NO

Pizza Log

DATE	
PIZZERIA	
NEIGHBORHOOD	

TOPPINGS

○ CHEESE	○ MUSHROOMS	○ ONIONS
○ PINEAPPLE	○ BACON	○ TUNA
○ GREEN PEPPER	○ SAUSAGE	○ BLACK OLIVES

○ OTHER

CHEESE

○ GREASY	○ STINGY
○ SMOKEY	○ STINKY
○ CREAMY	○ SALTY

SAUCE

○ SWEET	○ SAVORY
○ TANGY	○ SPICY
○ THIN	○ CHUNKY

CHEESE TO SAUCE RATIO (CSR)

CHEESE	☐ ☐ ☐ ☐ ☐ ☐
SAUCE	☐ ☐ ☐ ☐ ☐ ☐

FRESHNESS

○1 ○2 ○3 ○4 ○5

CRUST

CRUST SIZE	CRUST	
○ THIN	○ BUTTERY	○ CRISPY
○ MEDIUM	○ SPONGY	○ BUBBLY
○ LARGE	○ CHEWY	○ OTHER

CRUST

○1 ○2 ○3 ○4 ○5

STYLE	○ NY ○ CHICAGO ○ OTHER

COMMENTS

MY RATING	○1 ○2 ○3 ○4 ○5 ○6 ○7 ○8 ○9 ○10	EAT AGAIN?	○ YES ○ NO

Pizza Log

DATE	
PIZZERIA	
NEIGHBORHOOD	

TOPPINGS

○ CHEESE	○ MUSHROOMS	○ ONIONS
○ PINEAPPLE	○ BACON	○ TUNA
○ GREEN PEPPER	○ SAUSAGE	○ BLACK OLIVES
○ OTHER		

CHEESE

○ GREASY	○ STINGY
○ SMOKEY	○ STINKY
○ CREAMY	○ SALTY

SAUCE

○ SWEET	○ SAVORY
○ TANGY	○ SPICY
○ THIN	○ CHUNKY

CHEESE TO SAUCE RATIO (CSR)

CHEESE	☐☐☐☐☐☐
SAUCE	☐☐☐☐☐☐

FRESHNESS

○1 ○2 ○3 ○4 ○5

CRUST

CRUST SIZE	CRUST	
○ THIN	○ BUTTERY	○ CRISPY
○ MEDIUM	○ SPONGY	○ BUBBLY
○ LARGE	○ CHEWY	○ OTHER

CRUST

○1 ○2 ○3 ○4 ○5

STYLE	○ NY ○ CHICAGO ○ OTHER

COMMENTS

MY RATING	○1 ○2 ○3 ○4 ○5 ○6 ○7 ○8 ○9 ○10	EAT AGAIN?	○ YES ○ NO

Pizza Log

DATE	
PIZZERIA	
NEIGHBORHOOD	

TOPPINGS

- ○ CHEESE
- ○ MUSHROOMS
- ○ ONIONS
- ○ PINEAPPLE
- ○ BACON
- ○ TUNA
- ○ GREEN PEPPER
- ○ SAUSAGE
- ○ BLACK OLIVES
- ○ OTHER

CHEESE

- ○ GREASY
- ○ STINGY
- ○ SMOKEY
- ○ STINKY
- ○ CREAMY
- ○ SALTY

SAUCE

- ○ SWEET
- ○ SAVORY
- ○ TANGY
- ○ SPICY
- ○ THIN
- ○ CHUNKY

CHEESE TO SAUCE RATIO (CSR)

CHEESE	☐ ☐ ☐ ☐ ☐ ☐ ☐
SAUCE	☐ ☐ ☐ ☐ ☐ ☐ ☐

FRESHNESS

○ 1 ○ 2 ○ 3 ○ 4 ○ 5

CRUST SIZE

- ○ THIN
- ○ MEDIUM
- ○ LARGE

CRUST

- ○ BUTTERY
- ○ CRISPY
- ○ SPONGY
- ○ BUBBLY
- ○ CHEWY
- ○ OTHER

CRUST

○ 1 ○ 2 ○ 3 ○ 4 ○ 5

STYLE ○ NY ○ CHICAGO ○ OTHER

COMMENTS

MY RATING ○ 1 ○ 2 ○ 3 ○ 4 ○ 5 ○ 6 ○ 7 ○ 8 ○ 9 ○ 10

EAT AGAIN? ○ YES ○ NO

Pizza Log

DATE	
PIZZERIA	
NEIGHBORHOOD	

TOPPINGS

○ CHEESE	○ MUSHROOMS	○ ONIONS
○ PINEAPPLE	○ BACON	○ TUNA
○ GREEN PEPPER	○ SAUSAGE	○ BLACK OLIVES

○ OTHER

CHEESE

○ GREASY	○ STINGY
○ SMOKEY	○ STINKY
○ CREAMY	○ SALTY

SAUCE

○ SWEET	○ SAVORY
○ TANGY	○ SPICY
○ THIN	○ CHUNKY

CHEESE TO SAUCE RATIO (CSR)

CHEESE	☐☐☐☐☐☐
SAUCE	☐☐☐☐☐☐

FRESHNESS

○1 ○2 ○3 ○4 ○5

CRUST SIZE

○ THIN	
○ MEDIUM	
○ LARGE	

CRUST

○ BUTTERY	○ CRISPY
○ SPONGY	○ BUBBLY
○ CHEWY	○ OTHER

CRUST

○1 ○2 ○3 ○4 ○5

STYLE	○ NY ○ CHICAGO ○ OTHER

COMMENTS

MY RATING	○1 ○2 ○3 ○4 ○5 ○6 ○7 ○8 ○9 ○10	EAT AGAIN?	○ YES ○ NO

Pizza Log

DATE	
PIZZERIA	
NEIGHBORHOOD	

TOPPINGS

- ○ CHEESE
- ○ MUSHROOMS
- ○ ONIONS
- ○ PINEAPPLE
- ○ BACON
- ○ TUNA
- ○ GREEN PEPPER
- ○ SAUSAGE
- ○ BLACK OLIVES
- ○ OTHER

CHEESE

- ○ GREASY
- ○ STINGY
- ○ SMOKEY
- ○ STINKY
- ○ CREAMY
- ○ SALTY

SAUCE

- ○ SWEET
- ○ SAVORY
- ○ TANGY
- ○ SPICY
- ○ THIN
- ○ CHUNKY

CHEESE TO SAUCE RATIO (CSR)

CHEESE	☐☐☐☐☐☐
SAUCE	☐☐☐☐☐☐

FRESHNESS

○ 1　○ 2　○ 3　○ 4　○ 5

CRUST SIZE

- ○ THIN
- ○ MEDIUM
- ○ LARGE

CRUST

- ○ BUTTERY
- ○ CRISPY
- ○ SPONGY
- ○ BUBBLY
- ○ CHEWY
- ○ OTHER

CRUST

○ 1　○ 2　○ 3　○ 4　○ 5

STYLE ○ NY　○ CHICAGO　○ OTHER

COMMENTS

MY RATING ○ 1　○ 2　○ 3　○ 4　○ 5　○ 6　○ 7　○ 8　○ 9　○ 10

EAT AGAIN? ○ YES　○ NO

Pizza Log

DATE	
PIZZERIA	
NEIGHBORHOOD	

TOPPINGS

○ CHEESE	○ MUSHROOMS	○ ONIONS
○ PINEAPPLE	○ BACON	○ TUNA
○ GREEN PEPPER	○ SAUSAGE	○ BLACK OLIVES
○ OTHER		

CHEESE

○ GREASY	○ STINGY
○ SMOKEY	○ STINKY
○ CREAMY	○ SALTY

SAUCE

○ SWEET	○ SAVORY
○ TANGY	○ SPICY
○ THIN	○ CHUNKY

CHEESE TO SAUCE RATIO (CSR)

CHEESE	☐ ☐ ☐ ☐ ☐ ☐
SAUCE	☐ ☐ ☐ ☐ ☐ ☐

FRESHNESS

○1 ○2 ○3 ○4 ○5

CRUST SIZE

○ THIN	
○ MEDIUM	
○ LARGE	

CRUST

○ BUTTERY	○ CRISPY
○ SPONGY	○ BUBBLY
○ CHEWY	○ OTHER

CRUST

○1 ○2 ○3 ○4 ○5

STYLE	○ NY ○ CHICAGO ○ OTHER

COMMENTS

MY RATING	○1 ○2 ○3 ○4 ○5 ○6 ○7 ○8 ○9 ○10	EAT AGAIN?	○ YES ○ NO

Pizza Log

DATE	
PIZZERIA	
NEIGHBORHOOD	

TOPPINGS

○ CHEESE	○ MUSHROOMS	○ ONIONS
○ PINEAPPLE	○ BACON	○ TUNA
○ GREEN PEPPER	○ SAUSAGE	○ BLACK OLIVES
○ OTHER		

CHEESE

○ GREASY	○ STINGY
○ SMOKEY	○ STINKY
○ CREAMY	○ SALTY

SAUCE

○ SWEET	○ SAVORY
○ TANGY	○ SPICY
○ THIN	○ CHUNKY

CHEESE TO SAUCE RATIO (CSR)

CHEESE	☐☐☐☐☐☐
SAUCE	☐☐☐☐☐☐

FRESHNESS

○1 ○2 ○3 ○4 ○5

CRUST SIZE	CRUST		CRUST
○ THIN	○ BUTTERY	○ CRISPY	○1 ○2 ○3 ○4 ○5
○ MEDIUM	○ SPONGY	○ BUBBLY	
○ LARGE	○ CHEWY	○ OTHER	STYLE: ○ NY ○ CHICAGO ○ OTHER

COMMENTS

MY RATING	○1 ○2 ○3 ○4 ○5 ○6 ○7 ○8 ○9 ○10	EAT AGAIN?	○ YES ○ NO

Pizza Log

DATE	
PIZZERIA	
NEIGHBORHOOD	

TOPPINGS			CHEESE	
○ CHEESE	○ MUSHROOMS	○ ONIONS	○ GREASY	○ STINGY
○ PINEAPPLE	○ BACON	○ TUNA	○ SMOKEY	○ STINKY
○ GREEN PEPPER	○ SAUSAGE	○ BLACK OLIVES	○ CREAMY	○ SALTY
○ OTHER			SAUCE	
			○ SWEET	○ SAVORY
			○ TANGY	○ SPICY
			○ THIN	○ CHUNKY
			CHEESE TO SAUCE RATIO (CSR)	
FRESHNESS			CHEESE	☐☐☐☐☐☐
	○1 ○2 ○3 ○4 ○5		SAUCE	☐☐☐☐☐☐

CRUST SIZE	CRUST		CRUST	
○ THIN	○ BUTTERY	○ CRISPY	○1 ○2 ○3 ○4 ○5	
○ MEDIUM	○ SPONGY	○ BUBBLY		
○ LARGE	○ CHEWY	○ OTHER	STYLE	○ NY ○ CHICAGO ○ OTHER

COMMENTS

MY RATING	○1 ○2 ○3 ○4 ○5 ○6 ○7 ○8 ○9 ○10	EAT AGAIN?	○ YES ○ NO

Pizza Log

DATE	
PIZZERIA	
NEIGHBORHOOD	

TOPPINGS

○ CHEESE	○ MUSHROOMS	○ ONIONS
○ PINEAPPLE	○ BACON	○ TUNA
○ GREEN PEPPER	○ SAUSAGE	○ BLACK OLIVES
○ OTHER		

CHEESE

○ GREASY	○ STINGY
○ SMOKEY	○ STINKY
○ CREAMY	○ SALTY

SAUCE

○ SWEET	○ SAVORY
○ TANGY	○ SPICY
○ THIN	○ CHUNKY

CHEESE TO SAUCE RATIO (CSR)

CHEESE	☐ ☐ ☐ ☐ ☐ ☐
SAUCE	☐ ☐ ☐ ☐ ☐ ☐

FRESHNESS

○ 1 ○ 2 ○ 3 ○ 4 ○ 5

CRUST SIZE

○ THIN
○ MEDIUM
○ LARGE

CRUST

○ BUTTERY	○ CRISPY
○ SPONGY	○ BUBBLY
○ CHEWY	○ OTHER

CRUST

○ 1 ○ 2 ○ 3 ○ 4 ○ 5

STYLE	○ NY ○ CHICAGO ○ OTHER

COMMENTS

MY RATING	○ 1 ○ 2 ○ 3 ○ 4 ○ 5 ○ 6 ○ 7 ○ 8 ○ 9 ○ 10	EAT AGAIN?	○ YES ○ NO

Pizza Log

DATE	
PIZZERIA	
NEIGHBORHOOD	

TOPPINGS

○ CHEESE	○ MUSHROOMS	○ ONIONS
○ PINEAPPLE	○ BACON	○ TUNA
○ GREEN PEPPER	○ SAUSAGE	○ BLACK OLIVES
○ OTHER		

CHEESE

○ GREASY	○ STINGY
○ SMOKEY	○ STINKY
○ CREAMY	○ SALTY

SAUCE

○ SWEET	○ SAVORY
○ TANGY	○ SPICY
○ THIN	○ CHUNKY

CHEESE TO SAUCE RATIO (CSR)

CHEESE	☐☐☐☐☐☐
SAUCE	☐☐☐☐☐☐

FRESHNESS

○1 ○2 ○3 ○4 ○5

CRUST SIZE

○ THIN
○ MEDIUM
○ LARGE

CRUST

○ BUTTERY	○ CRISPY
○ SPONGY	○ BUBBLY
○ CHEWY	○ OTHER

CRUST

○1 ○2 ○3 ○4 ○5

STYLE	○ NY ○ CHICAGO ○ OTHER

COMMENTS

MY RATING	○1 ○2 ○3 ○4 ○5 ○6 ○7 ○8 ○9 ○10	EAT AGAIN?	○ YES ○ NO

Pizza Log

DATE	
PIZZERIA	
NEIGHBORHOOD	

TOPPINGS

○ CHEESE	○ MUSHROOMS	○ ONIONS
○ PINEAPPLE	○ BACON	○ TUNA
○ GREEN PEPPER	○ SAUSAGE	○ BLACK OLIVES
○ OTHER		

CHEESE

○ GREASY	○ STINGY
○ SMOKEY	○ STINKY
○ CREAMY	○ SALTY

SAUCE

○ SWEET	○ SAVORY
○ TANGY	○ SPICY
○ THIN	○ CHUNKY

CHEESE TO SAUCE RATIO (CSR)

CHEESE	☐☐☐☐☐☐
SAUCE	☐☐☐☐☐☐

FRESHNESS

○1 ○2 ○3 ○4 ○5

CRUST SIZE

○ THIN	
○ MEDIUM	
○ LARGE	

CRUST

○ BUTTERY	○ CRISPY
○ SPONGY	○ BUBBLY
○ CHEWY	○ OTHER

CRUST

○1 ○2 ○3 ○4 ○5

STYLE	○ NY ○ CHICAGO ○ OTHER

COMMENTS

MY RATING	○1 ○2 ○3 ○4 ○5 ○6 ○7 ○8 ○9 ○10	EAT AGAIN?	○ YES ○ NO

Pizza Log

DATE	
PIZZERIA	
NEIGHBORHOOD	

TOPPINGS

○ CHEESE	○ MUSHROOMS	○ ONIONS
○ PINEAPPLE	○ BACON	○ TUNA
○ GREEN PEPPER	○ SAUSAGE	○ BLACK OLIVES
○ OTHER		

CHEESE

○ GREASY	○ STINGY
○ SMOKEY	○ STINKY
○ CREAMY	○ SALTY

SAUCE

○ SWEET	○ SAVORY
○ TANGY	○ SPICY
○ THIN	○ CHUNKY

CHEESE TO SAUCE RATIO (CSR)

CHEESE	☐ ☐ ☐ ☐ ☐ ☐
SAUCE	☐ ☐ ☐ ☐ ☐ ☐

FRESHNESS

○ 1 ○ 2 ○ 3 ○ 4 ○ 5

CRUST SIZE / CRUST

CRUST SIZE	CRUST	
○ THIN	○ BUTTERY	○ CRISPY
○ MEDIUM	○ SPONGY	○ BUBBLY
○ LARGE	○ CHEWY	○ OTHER

CRUST

○ 1 ○ 2 ○ 3 ○ 4 ○ 5

STYLE	○ NY ○ CHICAGO ○ OTHER

COMMENTS

MY RATING	○ 1 ○ 2 ○ 3 ○ 4 ○ 5 ○ 6 ○ 7 ○ 8 ○ 9 ○ 10	EAT AGAIN?	○ YES ○ NO

Pizza Log

DATE	
PIZZERIA	
NEIGHBORHOOD	

TOPPINGS

- ○ CHEESE
- ○ MUSHROOMS
- ○ ONIONS
- ○ PINEAPPLE
- ○ BACON
- ○ TUNA
- ○ GREEN PEPPER
- ○ SAUSAGE
- ○ BLACK OLIVES
- ○ OTHER

CHEESE

- ○ GREASY
- ○ STINGY
- ○ SMOKEY
- ○ STINKY
- ○ CREAMY
- ○ SALTY

SAUCE

- ○ SWEET
- ○ SAVORY
- ○ TANGY
- ○ SPICY
- ○ THIN
- ○ CHUNKY

CHEESE TO SAUCE RATIO (CSR)

CHEESE	☐ ☐ ☐ ☐ ☐ ☐
SAUCE	☐ ☐ ☐ ☐ ☐ ☐

FRESHNESS

○ 1   ○ 2   ○ 3   ○ 4   ○ 5

CRUST SIZE

- ○ THIN
- ○ MEDIUM
- ○ LARGE

CRUST

- ○ BUTTERY
- ○ CRISPY
- ○ SPONGY
- ○ BUBBLY
- ○ CHEWY
- ○ OTHER

CRUST

○ 1   ○ 2   ○ 3   ○ 4   ○ 5

STYLE: ○ NY   ○ CHICAGO   ○ OTHER

COMMENTS

MY RATING: ○ 1   ○ 2   ○ 3   ○ 4   ○ 5   ○ 6   ○ 7   ○ 8   ○ 9   ○ 10

EAT AGAIN?: ○ YES   ○ NO

Pizza Log

DATE	
PIZZERIA	
NEIGHBORHOOD	

TOPPINGS

○ CHEESE	○ MUSHROOMS	○ ONIONS
○ PINEAPPLE	○ BACON	○ TUNA
○ GREEN PEPPER	○ SAUSAGE	○ BLACK OLIVES
○ OTHER		

CHEESE

○ GREASY	○ STINGY
○ SMOKEY	○ STINKY
○ CREAMY	○ SALTY

SAUCE

○ SWEET	○ SAVORY
○ TANGY	○ SPICY
○ THIN	○ CHUNKY

CHEESE TO SAUCE RATIO (CSR)

CHEESE	☐☐☐☐☐☐
SAUCE	☐☐☐☐☐☐

FRESHNESS

○ 1   ○ 2   ○ 3   ○ 4   ○ 5

CRUST

CRUST SIZE	CRUST	
○ THIN	○ BUTTERY	○ CRISPY
○ MEDIUM	○ SPONGY	○ BUBBLY
○ LARGE	○ CHEWY	○ OTHER

CRUST

○ 1   ○ 2   ○ 3   ○ 4   ○ 5

STYLE	○ NY ○ CHICAGO ○ OTHER

COMMENTS

MY RATING	○ 1 ○ 2 ○ 3 ○ 4 ○ 5 ○ 6 ○ 7 ○ 8 ○ 9 ○ 10	EAT AGAIN?	○ YES ○ NO

Pizza Log

DATE	
PIZZERIA	
NEIGHBORHOOD	

TOPPINGS

○ CHEESE	○ MUSHROOMS	○ ONIONS
○ PINEAPPLE	○ BACON	○ TUNA
○ GREEN PEPPER	○ SAUSAGE	○ BLACK OLIVES
○ OTHER		

CHEESE

○ GREASY	○ STINGY
○ SMOKEY	○ STINKY
○ CREAMY	○ SALTY

SAUCE

○ SWEET	○ SAVORY
○ TANGY	○ SPICY
○ THIN	○ CHUNKY

CHEESE TO SAUCE RATIO (CSR)

CHEESE	☐ ☐ ☐ ☐ ☐ ☐
SAUCE	☐ ☐ ☐ ☐ ☐ ☐

FRESHNESS

○1 ○2 ○3 ○4 ○5

CRUST

CRUST SIZE	CRUST		CRUST
○ THIN	○ BUTTERY	○ CRISPY	○1 ○2 ○3 ○4 ○5
○ MEDIUM	○ SPONGY	○ BUBBLY	
○ LARGE	○ CHEWY	○ OTHER	STYLE: ○ NY ○ CHICAGO ○ OTHER

COMMENTS

MY RATING	○1 ○2 ○3 ○4 ○5 ○6 ○7 ○8 ○9 ○10	EAT AGAIN?	○ YES ○ NO

Pizza Log

DATE	
PIZZERIA	
NEIGHBORHOOD	

TOPPINGS

○ CHEESE	○ MUSHROOMS	○ ONIONS
○ PINEAPPLE	○ BACON	○ TUNA
○ GREEN PEPPER	○ SAUSAGE	○ BLACK OLIVES
○ OTHER		

CHEESE

○ GREASY	○ STINGY
○ SMOKEY	○ STINKY
○ CREAMY	○ SALTY

SAUCE

○ SWEET	○ SAVORY
○ TANGY	○ SPICY
○ THIN	○ CHUNKY

CHEESE TO SAUCE RATIO (CSR)

CHEESE	☐☐☐☐☐☐
SAUCE	☐☐☐☐☐☐

FRESHNESS

○1 ○2 ○3 ○4 ○5

CRUST SIZE	CRUST	
○ THIN	○ BUTTERY	○ CRISPY
○ MEDIUM	○ SPONGY	○ BUBBLY
○ LARGE	○ CHEWY	○ OTHER

CRUST

○1 ○2 ○3 ○4 ○5

STYLE	○ NY ○ CHICAGO ○ OTHER

COMMENTS

MY RATING	○1 ○2 ○3 ○4 ○5 ○6 ○7 ○8 ○9 ○10	EAT AGAIN?	○ YES ○ NO

Pizza Log

DATE	
PIZZERIA	
NEIGHBORHOOD	

TOPPINGS			CHEESE	
○ CHEESE	○ MUSHROOMS	○ ONIONS	○ GREASY	○ STINGY
○ PINEAPPLE	○ BACON	○ TUNA	○ SMOKEY	○ STINKY
○ GREEN PEPPER	○ SAUSAGE	○ BLACK OLIVES	○ CREAMY	○ SALTY
○ OTHER			**SAUCE**	
			○ SWEET	○ SAVORY
			○ TANGY	○ SPICY
			○ THIN	○ CHUNKY
			CHEESE TO SAUCE RATIO (CSR)	
FRESHNESS			CHEESE	☐☐☐☐☐☐
○1 ○2 ○3 ○4 ○5			SAUCE	☐☐☐☐☐☐

CRUST SIZE	CRUST		CRUST	
○ THIN	○ BUTTERY	○ CRISPY	○1 ○2 ○3 ○4 ○5	
○ MEDIUM	○ SPONGY	○ BUBBLY		
○ LARGE	○ CHEWY	○ OTHER	STYLE	○ NY ○ CHICAGO ○ OTHER

COMMENTS

MY RATING	○1 ○2 ○3 ○4 ○5 ○6 ○7 ○8 ○9 ○10	EAT AGAIN?	○ YES ○ NO

Pizza Log

DATE	
PIZZERIA	
NEIGHBORHOOD	

TOPPINGS			CHEESE	
○ CHEESE	○ MUSHROOMS	○ ONIONS	○ GREASY	○ STINGY
○ PINEAPPLE	○ BACON	○ TUNA	○ SMOKEY	○ STINKY
○ GREEN PEPPER	○ SAUSAGE	○ BLACK OLIVES	○ CREAMY	○ SALTY

○ OTHER			SAUCE	
			○ SWEET	○ SAVORY
			○ TANGY	○ SPICY
			○ THIN	○ CHUNKY

			CHEESE TO SAUCE RATIO (CSR)	
FRESHNESS			CHEESE	☐☐☐☐☐☐
○1 ○2 ○3 ○4 ○5			SAUCE	☐☐☐☐☐☐

CRUST SIZE	CRUST		CRUST	
○ THIN	○ BUTTERY	○ CRISPY	○1 ○2 ○3 ○4 ○5	
○ MEDIUM	○ SPONGY	○ BUBBLY		
○ LARGE	○ CHEWY	○ OTHER	STYLE	○ NY ○ CHICAGO ○ OTHER

COMMENTS

MY RATING	○1 ○2 ○3 ○4 ○5 ○6 ○7 ○8 ○9 ○10	EAT AGAIN?	○ YES ○ NO

Pizza Log

DATE	
PIZZERIA	
NEIGHBORHOOD	

TOPPINGS

○ CHEESE	○ MUSHROOMS	○ ONIONS
○ PINEAPPLE	○ BACON	○ TUNA
○ GREEN PEPPER	○ SAUSAGE	○ BLACK OLIVES
○ OTHER		

CHEESE

○ GREASY	○ STINGY
○ SMOKEY	○ STINKY
○ CREAMY	○ SALTY

SAUCE

○ SWEET	○ SAVORY
○ TANGY	○ SPICY
○ THIN	○ CHUNKY

CHEESE TO SAUCE RATIO (CSR)

CHEESE	☐☐☐☐☐☐☐
SAUCE	☐☐☐☐☐☐☐

FRESHNESS

○1 ○2 ○3 ○4 ○5

CRUST

CRUST SIZE	CRUST	
○ THIN	○ BUTTERY	○ CRISPY
○ MEDIUM	○ SPONGY	○ BUBBLY
○ LARGE	○ CHEWY	○ OTHER

CRUST

○1 ○2 ○3 ○4 ○5

STYLE	○ NY ○ CHICAGO ○ OTHER

COMMENTS

MY RATING	○1 ○2 ○3 ○4 ○5 ○6 ○7 ○8 ○9 ○10	EAT AGAIN?	○ YES ○ NO

Pizza Log

DATE	
PIZZERIA	
NEIGHBORHOOD	

TOPPINGS

○ CHEESE	○ MUSHROOMS	○ ONIONS
○ PINEAPPLE	○ BACON	○ TUNA
○ GREEN PEPPER	○ SAUSAGE	○ BLACK OLIVES
○ OTHER		

CHEESE

○ GREASY	○ STINGY
○ SMOKEY	○ STINKY
○ CREAMY	○ SALTY

SAUCE

○ SWEET	○ SAVORY
○ TANGY	○ SPICY
○ THIN	○ CHUNKY

CHEESE TO SAUCE RATIO (CSR)

CHEESE	☐☐☐☐☐☐
SAUCE	☐☐☐☐☐☐

FRESHNESS

○1 ○2 ○3 ○4 ○5

CRUST SIZE

○ THIN	
○ MEDIUM	
○ LARGE	

CRUST

○ BUTTERY	○ CRISPY
○ SPONGY	○ BUBBLY
○ CHEWY	○ OTHER

CRUST

○1 ○2 ○3 ○4 ○5

STYLE	○ NY ○ CHICAGO ○ OTHER

COMMENTS

MY RATING	○1 ○2 ○3 ○4 ○5 ○6 ○7 ○8 ○9 ○10	EAT AGAIN?	○ YES ○ NO

Pizza Log

DATE	
PIZZERIA	
NEIGHBORHOOD	

TOPPINGS

○ CHEESE	○ MUSHROOMS	○ ONIONS
○ PINEAPPLE	○ BACON	○ TUNA
○ GREEN PEPPER	○ SAUSAGE	○ BLACK OLIVES
○ OTHER		

CHEESE

○ GREASY	○ STINGY
○ SMOKEY	○ STINKY
○ CREAMY	○ SALTY

SAUCE

○ SWEET	○ SAVORY
○ TANGY	○ SPICY
○ THIN	○ CHUNKY

CHEESE TO SAUCE RATIO (CSR)

CHEESE	☐☐☐☐☐☐
SAUCE	☐☐☐☐☐☐

FRESHNESS

○1 ○2 ○3 ○4 ○5

CRUST

CRUST SIZE	CRUST	
○ THIN	○ BUTTERY	○ CRISPY
○ MEDIUM	○ SPONGY	○ BUBBLY
○ LARGE	○ CHEWY	○ OTHER

CRUST

○1 ○2 ○3 ○4 ○5

STYLE	○ NY ○ CHICAGO ○ OTHER

COMMENTS

MY RATING	○1 ○2 ○3 ○4 ○5 ○6 ○7 ○8 ○9 ○10	EAT AGAIN?	○ YES ○ NO

Pizza Log

DATE	
PIZZERIA	
NEIGHBORHOOD	

TOPPINGS

○ CHEESE	○ MUSHROOMS	○ ONIONS
○ PINEAPPLE	○ BACON	○ TUNA
○ GREEN PEPPER	○ SAUSAGE	○ BLACK OLIVES
○ OTHER		

CHEESE

○ GREASY	○ STINGY
○ SMOKEY	○ STINKY
○ CREAMY	○ SALTY

SAUCE

○ SWEET	○ SAVORY
○ TANGY	○ SPICY
○ THIN	○ CHUNKY

CHEESE TO SAUCE RATIO (CSR)

CHEESE	☐ ☐ ☐ ☐ ☐ ☐
SAUCE	☐ ☐ ☐ ☐ ☐ ☐

FRESHNESS

○1 ○2 ○3 ○4 ○5

CRUST

CRUST SIZE	CRUST	
○ THIN	○ BUTTERY	○ CRISPY
○ MEDIUM	○ SPONGY	○ BUBBLY
○ LARGE	○ CHEWY	○ OTHER

CRUST

○1 ○2 ○3 ○4 ○5

STYLE	○ NY ○ CHICAGO ○ OTHER

COMMENTS

MY RATING	○1 ○2 ○3 ○4 ○5 ○6 ○7 ○8 ○9 ○10	EAT AGAIN?	○ YES ○ NO

Pizza Log

DATE	
PIZZERIA	
NEIGHBORHOOD	

TOPPINGS

- ○ CHEESE
- ○ MUSHROOMS
- ○ ONIONS
- ○ PINEAPPLE
- ○ BACON
- ○ TUNA
- ○ GREEN PEPPER
- ○ SAUSAGE
- ○ BLACK OLIVES
- ○ OTHER

CHEESE

- ○ GREASY
- ○ STINGY
- ○ SMOKEY
- ○ STINKY
- ○ CREAMY
- ○ SALTY

SAUCE

- ○ SWEET
- ○ SAVORY
- ○ TANGY
- ○ SPICY
- ○ THIN
- ○ CHUNKY

CHEESE TO SAUCE RATIO (CSR)

CHEESE	☐☐☐☐☐☐
SAUCE	☐☐☐☐☐☐

FRESHNESS

○ 1 ○ 2 ○ 3 ○ 4 ○ 5

CRUST SIZE

- ○ THIN
- ○ MEDIUM
- ○ LARGE

CRUST

- ○ BUTTERY
- ○ CRISPY
- ○ SPONGY
- ○ BUBBLY
- ○ CHEWY
- ○ OTHER

CRUST

○ 1 ○ 2 ○ 3 ○ 4 ○ 5

STYLE	○ NY ○ CHICAGO ○ OTHER

COMMENTS

MY RATING: ○ 1 ○ 2 ○ 3 ○ 4 ○ 5 ○ 6 ○ 7 ○ 8 ○ 9 ○ 10

EAT AGAIN?: ○ YES ○ NO

Pizza Log

DATE	
PIZZERIA	
NEIGHBORHOOD	

TOPPINGS

○ CHEESE	○ MUSHROOMS	○ ONIONS
○ PINEAPPLE	○ BACON	○ TUNA
○ GREEN PEPPER	○ SAUSAGE	○ BLACK OLIVES

○ OTHER

CHEESE

○ GREASY	○ STINGY
○ SMOKEY	○ STINKY
○ CREAMY	○ SALTY

SAUCE

○ SWEET	○ SAVORY
○ TANGY	○ SPICY
○ THIN	○ CHUNKY

FRESHNESS

○ 1 ○ 2 ○ 3 ○ 4 ○ 5

CHEESE TO SAUCE RATIO (CSR)

CHEESE	☐ ☐ ☐ ☐ ☐ ☐
SAUCE	☐ ☐ ☐ ☐ ☐ ☐

CRUST SIZE

○ THIN
○ MEDIUM
○ LARGE

CRUST

○ BUTTERY	○ CRISPY
○ SPONGY	○ BUBBLY
○ CHEWY	○ OTHER

CRUST

○ 1 ○ 2 ○ 3 ○ 4 ○ 5

STYLE	○ NY ○ CHICAGO ○ OTHER

COMMENTS

MY RATING	○ 1 ○ 2 ○ 3 ○ 4 ○ 5 ○ 6 ○ 7 ○ 8 ○ 9 ○ 10	EAT AGAIN?	○ YES ○ NO

Pizza Log

DATE	
PIZZERIA	
NEIGHBORHOOD	

TOPPINGS

○ CHEESE	○ MUSHROOMS	○ ONIONS
○ PINEAPPLE	○ BACON	○ TUNA
○ GREEN PEPPER	○ SAUSAGE	○ BLACK OLIVES
○ OTHER		

CHEESE

○ GREASY	○ STINGY
○ SMOKEY	○ STINKY
○ CREAMY	○ SALTY

SAUCE

○ SWEET	○ SAVORY
○ TANGY	○ SPICY
○ THIN	○ CHUNKY

CHEESE TO SAUCE RATIO (CSR)

CHEESE	☐ ☐ ☐ ☐ ☐ ☐
SAUCE	☐ ☐ ☐ ☐ ☐ ☐

FRESHNESS

○1　○2　○3　○4　○5

CRUST SIZE	CRUST		CRUST
○ THIN	○ BUTTERY	○ CRISPY	○1　○2　○3　○4　○5
○ MEDIUM	○ SPONGY	○ BUBBLY	
○ LARGE	○ CHEWY	○ OTHER	STYLE: ○ NY　○ CHICAGO　○ OTHER

COMMENTS

MY RATING	○1 ○2 ○3 ○4 ○5 ○6 ○7 ○8 ○9 ○10
EAT AGAIN?	○ YES　○ NO

Pizza Log

DATE	
PIZZERIA	
NEIGHBORHOOD	

TOPPINGS

○ CHEESE	○ MUSHROOMS	○ ONIONS
○ PINEAPPLE	○ BACON	○ TUNA
○ GREEN PEPPER	○ SAUSAGE	○ BLACK OLIVES
○ OTHER		

CHEESE

○ GREASY	○ STINGY
○ SMOKEY	○ STINKY
○ CREAMY	○ SALTY

SAUCE

○ SWEET	○ SAVORY
○ TANGY	○ SPICY
○ THIN	○ CHUNKY

CHEESE TO SAUCE RATIO (CSR)

CHEESE	☐☐☐☐☐☐
SAUCE	☐☐☐☐☐☐

FRESHNESS
○1 ○2 ○3 ○4 ○5

CRUST SIZE	CRUST		CRUST	
○ THIN	○ BUTTERY	○ CRISPY	○1 ○2 ○3 ○4 ○5	
○ MEDIUM	○ SPONGY	○ BUBBLY	STYLE	○ NY ○ CHICAGO ○ OTHER
○ LARGE	○ CHEWY	○ OTHER		

COMMENTS

MY RATING	○1 ○2 ○3 ○4 ○5 ○6 ○7 ○8 ○9 ○10	EAT AGAIN?	○ YES ○ NO

Pizza Log

DATE	
PIZZERIA	
NEIGHBORHOOD	

TOPPINGS

○ CHEESE	○ MUSHROOMS	○ ONIONS
○ PINEAPPLE	○ BACON	○ TUNA
○ GREEN PEPPER	○ SAUSAGE	○ BLACK OLIVES
○ OTHER		

CHEESE

○ GREASY	○ STINGY
○ SMOKEY	○ STINKY
○ CREAMY	○ SALTY

SAUCE

○ SWEET	○ SAVORY
○ TANGY	○ SPICY
○ THIN	○ CHUNKY

CHEESE TO SAUCE RATIO (CSR)

CHEESE	☐ ☐ ☐ ☐ ☐ ☐
SAUCE	☐ ☐ ☐ ☐ ☐ ☐

FRESHNESS

○1　○2　○3　○4　○5

CRUST SIZE

○ THIN	
○ MEDIUM	
○ LARGE	

CRUST

○ BUTTERY	○ CRISPY
○ SPONGY	○ BUBBLY
○ CHEWY	○ OTHER

CRUST

○1　○2　○3　○4　○5

STYLE	○ NY ○ CHICAGO ○ OTHER

COMMENTS

MY RATING	○1 ○2 ○3 ○4 ○5 ○6 ○7 ○8 ○9 ○10	EAT AGAIN?	○ YES ○ NO

Pizza Log

DATE	
PIZZERIA	
NEIGHBORHOOD	

TOPPINGS			CHEESE	
○ CHEESE	○ MUSHROOMS	○ ONIONS	○ GREASY	○ STINGY
○ PINEAPPLE	○ BACON	○ TUNA	○ SMOKEY	○ STINKY
○ GREEN PEPPER	○ SAUSAGE	○ BLACK OLIVES	○ CREAMY	○ SALTY

OTHER		SAUCE	
○ OTHER		○ SWEET	○ SAVORY
		○ TANGY	○ SPICY
		○ THIN	○ CHUNKY

	CHEESE TO SAUCE RATIO (CSR)
CHEESE	☐☐☐☐☐☐
SAUCE	☐☐☐☐☐☐

FRESHNESS
○ 1   ○ 2   ○ 3   ○ 4   ○ 5

CRUST SIZE	CRUST		CRUST
○ THIN	○ BUTTERY	○ CRISPY	○ 1 ○ 2 ○ 3 ○ 4 ○ 5
○ MEDIUM	○ SPONGY	○ BUBBLY	
○ LARGE	○ CHEWY	○ OTHER	STYLE: ○ NY ○ CHICAGO ○ OTHER

COMMENTS

MY RATING	○1 ○2 ○3 ○4 ○5 ○6 ○7 ○8 ○9 ○10	EAT AGAIN?	○ YES ○ NO

Pizza Log

DATE	
PIZZERIA	
NEIGHBORHOOD	

TOPPINGS

○ CHEESE	○ MUSHROOMS	○ ONIONS
○ PINEAPPLE	○ BACON	○ TUNA
○ GREEN PEPPER	○ SAUSAGE	○ BLACK OLIVES
○ OTHER		

CHEESE

○ GREASY	○ STINGY
○ SMOKEY	○ STINKY
○ CREAMY	○ SALTY

SAUCE

○ SWEET	○ SAVORY
○ TANGY	○ SPICY
○ THIN	○ CHUNKY

CHEESE TO SAUCE RATIO (CSR)

CHEESE	☐ ☐ ☐ ☐ ☐ ☐
SAUCE	☐ ☐ ☐ ☐ ☐ ☐

FRESHNESS

○1 ○2 ○3 ○4 ○5

CRUST SIZE	CRUST		CRUST
○ THIN	○ BUTTERY	○ CRISPY	○1 ○2 ○3 ○4 ○5
○ MEDIUM	○ SPONGY	○ BUBBLY	
○ LARGE	○ CHEWY	○ OTHER	STYLE: ○ NY ○ CHICAGO ○ OTHER

COMMENTS

MY RATING	○1 ○2 ○3 ○4 ○5 ○6 ○7 ○8 ○9 ○10	EAT AGAIN?	○ YES ○ NO

Pizza Log

DATE	
PIZZERIA	
NEIGHBORHOOD	

TOPPINGS

○ CHEESE	○ MUSHROOMS	○ ONIONS
○ PINEAPPLE	○ BACON	○ TUNA
○ GREEN PEPPER	○ SAUSAGE	○ BLACK OLIVES
○ OTHER		

CHEESE

○ GREASY	○ STINGY
○ SMOKEY	○ STINKY
○ CREAMY	○ SALTY

SAUCE

○ SWEET	○ SAVORY
○ TANGY	○ SPICY
○ THIN	○ CHUNKY

CHEESE TO SAUCE RATIO (CSR)

CHEESE	☐☐☐☐☐☐
SAUCE	☐☐☐☐☐☐

FRESHNESS

○1　○2　○3　○4　○5

CRUST SIZE

○ THIN	
○ MEDIUM	
○ LARGE	

CRUST

○ BUTTERY	○ CRISPY
○ SPONGY	○ BUBBLY
○ CHEWY	○ OTHER

CRUST

○1　○2　○3　○4　○5

STYLE	○ NY　○ CHICAGO　○ OTHER

COMMENTS

MY RATING	○1 ○2 ○3 ○4 ○5 ○6 ○7 ○8 ○9 ○10	EAT AGAIN?	○ YES ○ NO

Pizza Log

DATE	
PIZZERIA	
NEIGHBORHOOD	

TOPPINGS

○ CHEESE	○ MUSHROOMS	○ ONIONS
○ PINEAPPLE	○ BACON	○ TUNA
○ GREEN PEPPER	○ SAUSAGE	○ BLACK OLIVES
○ OTHER		

CHEESE

○ GREASY	○ STINGY
○ SMOKEY	○ STINKY
○ CREAMY	○ SALTY

SAUCE

○ SWEET	○ SAVORY
○ TANGY	○ SPICY
○ THIN	○ CHUNKY

CHEESE TO SAUCE RATIO (CSR)

CHEESE	☐☐☐☐☐☐
SAUCE	☐☐☐☐☐☐

FRESHNESS

○1 ○2 ○3 ○4 ○5

CRUST

CRUST SIZE	CRUST		CRUST
○ THIN	○ BUTTERY	○ CRISPY	○1 ○2 ○3 ○4 ○5
○ MEDIUM	○ SPONGY	○ BUBBLY	
○ LARGE	○ CHEWY	○ OTHER	STYLE: ○ NY ○ CHICAGO ○ OTHER

COMMENTS

MY RATING	○1 ○2 ○3 ○4 ○5 ○6 ○7 ○8 ○9 ○10	EAT AGAIN?	○ YES ○ NO

Pizza Log

DATE	
PIZZERIA	
NEIGHBORHOOD	

TOPPINGS

○ CHEESE	○ MUSHROOMS	○ ONIONS
○ PINEAPPLE	○ BACON	○ TUNA
○ GREEN PEPPER	○ SAUSAGE	○ BLACK OLIVES
○ OTHER		

CHEESE

○ GREASY	○ STINGY
○ SMOKEY	○ STINKY
○ CREAMY	○ SALTY

SAUCE

○ SWEET	○ SAVORY
○ TANGY	○ SPICY
○ THIN	○ CHUNKY

CHEESE TO SAUCE RATIO (CSR)

CHEESE	☐☐☐☐☐☐
SAUCE	☐☐☐☐☐☐

FRESHNESS

○1 ○2 ○3 ○4 ○5

CRUST

CRUST SIZE	CRUST	
○ THIN	○ BUTTERY	○ CRISPY
○ MEDIUM	○ SPONGY	○ BUBBLY
○ LARGE	○ CHEWY	○ OTHER

CRUST

○1 ○2 ○3 ○4 ○5

STYLE	○ NY ○ CHICAGO ○ OTHER

COMMENTS

MY RATING	○1 ○2 ○3 ○4 ○5 ○6 ○7 ○8 ○9 ○10	EAT AGAIN?	○ YES ○ NO

Pizza Log

DATE	
PIZZERIA	
NEIGHBORHOOD	

TOPPINGS

○ CHEESE	○ MUSHROOMS	○ ONIONS
○ PINEAPPLE	○ BACON	○ TUNA
○ GREEN PEPPER	○ SAUSAGE	○ BLACK OLIVES
○ OTHER		

CHEESE

○ GREASY	○ STINGY
○ SMOKEY	○ STINKY
○ CREAMY	○ SALTY

SAUCE

○ SWEET	○ SAVORY
○ TANGY	○ SPICY
○ THIN	○ CHUNKY

FRESHNESS

○ 1   ○ 2   ○ 3   ○ 4   ○ 5

CHEESE TO SAUCE RATIO (CSR)

CHEESE	☐ ☐ ☐ ☐ ☐ ☐
SAUCE	☐ ☐ ☐ ☐ ☐ ☐

CRUST SIZE / CRUST

CRUST SIZE	CRUST	
○ THIN	○ BUTTERY	○ CRISPY
○ MEDIUM	○ SPONGY	○ BUBBLY
○ LARGE	○ CHEWY	○ OTHER

CRUST

○ 1   ○ 2   ○ 3   ○ 4   ○ 5

STYLE: ○ NY ○ CHICAGO ○ OTHER

COMMENTS

MY RATING: ○ 1 ○ 2 ○ 3 ○ 4 ○ 5 ○ 6 ○ 7 ○ 8 ○ 9 ○ 10

EAT AGAIN?: ○ YES ○ NO

Pizza Log

DATE	
PIZZERIA	
NEIGHBORHOOD	

TOPPINGS			CHEESE	
○ CHEESE	○ MUSHROOMS	○ ONIONS	○ GREASY	○ STINGY
○ PINEAPPLE	○ BACON	○ TUNA	○ SMOKEY	○ STINKY
○ GREEN PEPPER	○ SAUSAGE	○ BLACK OLIVES	○ CREAMY	○ SALTY
○ OTHER			SAUCE	
			○ SWEET	○ SAVORY
			○ TANGY	○ SPICY
			○ THIN	○ CHUNKY
			CHEESE TO SAUCE RATIO (CSR)	
FRESHNESS			CHEESE	☐☐☐☐☐☐
	○1 ○2 ○3 ○4 ○5		SAUCE	☐☐☐☐☐☐

CRUST SIZE	CRUST		CRUST	
○ THIN	○ BUTTERY	○ CRISPY	○1 ○2 ○3 ○4 ○5	
○ MEDIUM	○ SPONGY	○ BUBBLY	STYLE	○ NY ○ CHICAGO ○ OTHER
○ LARGE	○ CHEWY	○ OTHER		

COMMENTS

MY RATING	○1 ○2 ○3 ○4 ○5 ○6 ○7 ○8 ○9 ○10	EAT AGAIN?	○ YES ○ NO

Pizza Log

DATE	
PIZZERIA	
NEIGHBORHOOD	

TOPPINGS

○ CHEESE	○ MUSHROOMS	○ ONIONS
○ PINEAPPLE	○ BACON	○ TUNA
○ GREEN PEPPER	○ SAUSAGE	○ BLACK OLIVES
○ OTHER		

CHEESE

○ GREASY	○ STINGY
○ SMOKEY	○ STINKY
○ CREAMY	○ SALTY

SAUCE

○ SWEET	○ SAVORY
○ TANGY	○ SPICY
○ THIN	○ CHUNKY

CHEESE TO SAUCE RATIO (CSR)

CHEESE	☐☐☐☐☐☐☐
SAUCE	☐☐☐☐☐☐☐

FRESHNESS

○1 ○2 ○3 ○4 ○5

CRUST

CRUST SIZE	CRUST	
○ THIN	○ BUTTERY	○ CRISPY
○ MEDIUM	○ SPONGY	○ BUBBLY
○ LARGE	○ CHEWY	○ OTHER

CRUST

○1 ○2 ○3 ○4 ○5

STYLE	○ NY ○ CHICAGO ○ OTHER

COMMENTS

MY RATING	○1 ○2 ○3 ○4 ○5 ○6 ○7 ○8 ○9 ○10	EAT AGAIN?	○ YES ○ NO

Pizza Log

DATE	
PIZZERIA	
NEIGHBORHOOD	

TOPPINGS

○ CHEESE	○ MUSHROOMS	○ ONIONS
○ PINEAPPLE	○ BACON	○ TUNA
○ GREEN PEPPER	○ SAUSAGE	○ BLACK OLIVES
○ OTHER		

CHEESE

○ GREASY	○ STINGY
○ SMOKEY	○ STINKY
○ CREAMY	○ SALTY

SAUCE

○ SWEET	○ SAVORY
○ TANGY	○ SPICY
○ THIN	○ CHUNKY

CHEESE TO SAUCE RATIO (CSR)

CHEESE	☐ ☐ ☐ ☐ ☐ ☐
SAUCE	☐ ☐ ☐ ☐ ☐ ☐

FRESHNESS

○ 1 ○ 2 ○ 3 ○ 4 ○ 5

CRUST SIZE

○ THIN	
○ MEDIUM	
○ LARGE	

CRUST

○ BUTTERY	○ CRISPY
○ SPONGY	○ BUBBLY
○ CHEWY	○ OTHER

CRUST

○ 1 ○ 2 ○ 3 ○ 4 ○ 5

STYLE	○ NY ○ CHICAGO ○ OTHER

COMMENTS

MY RATING	○ 1 ○ 2 ○ 3 ○ 4 ○ 5 ○ 6 ○ 7 ○ 8 ○ 9 ○ 10	EAT AGAIN?	○ YES ○ NO

Pizza Log

DATE	
PIZZERIA	
NEIGHBORHOOD	

TOPPINGS

○ CHEESE	○ MUSHROOMS	○ ONIONS
○ PINEAPPLE	○ BACON	○ TUNA
○ GREEN PEPPER	○ SAUSAGE	○ BLACK OLIVES
○ OTHER		

CHEESE

○ GREASY	○ STINGY
○ SMOKEY	○ STINKY
○ CREAMY	○ SALTY

SAUCE

○ SWEET	○ SAVORY
○ TANGY	○ SPICY
○ THIN	○ CHUNKY

CHEESE TO SAUCE RATIO (CSR)

CHEESE	☐☐☐☐☐☐
SAUCE	☐☐☐☐☐☐

FRESHNESS

○1 ○2 ○3 ○4 ○5

CRUST SIZE

- ○ THIN
- ○ MEDIUM
- ○ LARGE

CRUST

○ BUTTERY	○ CRISPY
○ SPONGY	○ BUBBLY
○ CHEWY	○ OTHER

CRUST

○1 ○2 ○3 ○4 ○5

STYLE	○ NY ○ CHICAGO ○ OTHER

COMMENTS

MY RATING	○1 ○2 ○3 ○4 ○5 ○6 ○7 ○8 ○9 ○10	EAT AGAIN?	○ YES ○ NO

Pizza Log

DATE	
PIZZERIA	
NEIGHBORHOOD	

TOPPINGS

○ CHEESE	○ MUSHROOMS	○ ONIONS
○ PINEAPPLE	○ BACON	○ TUNA
○ GREEN PEPPER	○ SAUSAGE	○ BLACK OLIVES
○ OTHER		

CHEESE

○ GREASY	○ STINGY
○ SMOKEY	○ STINKY
○ CREAMY	○ SALTY

SAUCE

○ SWEET	○ SAVORY
○ TANGY	○ SPICY
○ THIN	○ CHUNKY

CHEESE TO SAUCE RATIO (CSR)

CHEESE	☐☐☐☐☐☐
SAUCE	☐☐☐☐☐☐

FRESHNESS

○1 ○2 ○3 ○4 ○5

CRUST SIZE	CRUST	
○ THIN	○ BUTTERY	○ CRISPY
○ MEDIUM	○ SPONGY	○ BUBBLY
○ LARGE	○ CHEWY	○ OTHER

CRUST

○1 ○2 ○3 ○4 ○5

STYLE	○ NY ○ CHICAGO ○ OTHER

COMMENTS

MY RATING	○1 ○2 ○3 ○4 ○5 ○6 ○7 ○8 ○9 ○10	EAT AGAIN?	○ YES ○ NO

Pizza Log

DATE	
PIZZERIA	
NEIGHBORHOOD	

TOPPINGS

○ CHEESE	○ MUSHROOMS	○ ONIONS
○ PINEAPPLE	○ BACON	○ TUNA
○ GREEN PEPPER	○ SAUSAGE	○ BLACK OLIVES
○ OTHER		

CHEESE

○ GREASY	○ STINGY
○ SMOKEY	○ STINKY
○ CREAMY	○ SALTY

SAUCE

○ SWEET	○ SAVORY
○ TANGY	○ SPICY
○ THIN	○ CHUNKY

CHEESE TO SAUCE RATIO (CSR)

CHEESE	☐ ☐ ☐ ☐ ☐ ☐
SAUCE	☐ ☐ ☐ ☐ ☐ ☐

FRESHNESS

○ 1 ○ 2 ○ 3 ○ 4 ○ 5

CRUST SIZE	CRUST	
○ THIN	○ BUTTERY	○ CRISPY
○ MEDIUM	○ SPONGY	○ BUBBLY
○ LARGE	○ CHEWY	○ OTHER

CRUST

○ 1 ○ 2 ○ 3 ○ 4 ○ 5

STYLE	○ NY ○ CHICAGO ○ OTHER

COMMENTS

MY RATING	○ 1 ○ 2 ○ 3 ○ 4 ○ 5 ○ 6 ○ 7 ○ 8 ○ 9 ○ 10	EAT AGAIN?	○ YES ○ NO

Pizza Log

DATE	
PIZZERIA	
NEIGHBORHOOD	

TOPPINGS

○ CHEESE	○ MUSHROOMS	○ ONIONS
○ PINEAPPLE	○ BACON	○ TUNA
○ GREEN PEPPER	○ SAUSAGE	○ BLACK OLIVES
○ OTHER		

CHEESE

○ GREASY	○ STINGY
○ SMOKEY	○ STINKY
○ CREAMY	○ SALTY

SAUCE

○ SWEET	○ SAVORY
○ TANGY	○ SPICY
○ THIN	○ CHUNKY

CHEESE TO SAUCE RATIO (CSR)

CHEESE	☐ ☐ ☐ ☐ ☐ ☐
SAUCE	☐ ☐ ☐ ☐ ☐ ☐

FRESHNESS

○1 ○2 ○3 ○4 ○5

CRUST SIZE

○ THIN	
○ MEDIUM	
○ LARGE	

CRUST

○ BUTTERY	○ CRISPY
○ SPONGY	○ BUBBLY
○ CHEWY	○ OTHER

CRUST

○1 ○2 ○3 ○4 ○5

STYLE	○ NY ○ CHICAGO ○ OTHER

COMMENTS

MY RATING	○1 ○2 ○3 ○4 ○5 ○6 ○7 ○8 ○9 ○10	EAT AGAIN?	○ YES ○ NO

Pizza Log

DATE	
PIZZERIA	
NEIGHBORHOOD	

TOPPINGS

○ CHEESE	○ MUSHROOMS	○ ONIONS
○ PINEAPPLE	○ BACON	○ TUNA
○ GREEN PEPPER	○ SAUSAGE	○ BLACK OLIVES
○ OTHER		

CHEESE

○ GREASY	○ STINGY
○ SMOKEY	○ STINKY
○ CREAMY	○ SALTY

SAUCE

○ SWEET	○ SAVORY
○ TANGY	○ SPICY
○ THIN	○ CHUNKY

CHEESE TO SAUCE RATIO (CSR)

CHEESE	☐ ☐ ☐ ☐ ☐ ☐ ☐
SAUCE	☐ ☐ ☐ ☐ ☐ ☐ ☐

FRESHNESS

○1 ○2 ○3 ○4 ○5

CRUST SIZE	CRUST		CRUST
○ THIN	○ BUTTERY	○ CRISPY	○1 ○2 ○3 ○4 ○5
○ MEDIUM	○ SPONGY	○ BUBBLY	
○ LARGE	○ CHEWY	○ OTHER	STYLE: ○ NY ○ CHICAGO ○ OTHER

COMMENTS

MY RATING	○1 ○2 ○3 ○4 ○5 ○6 ○7 ○8 ○9 ○10	EAT AGAIN?	○ YES ○ NO

Pizza Log

DATE	
PIZZERIA	
NEIGHBORHOOD	

TOPPINGS

○ CHEESE	○ MUSHROOMS	○ ONIONS
○ PINEAPPLE	○ BACON	○ TUNA
○ GREEN PEPPER	○ SAUSAGE	○ BLACK OLIVES

○ OTHER

CHEESE

○ GREASY	○ STINGY
○ SMOKEY	○ STINKY
○ CREAMY	○ SALTY

SAUCE

○ SWEET	○ SAVORY
○ TANGY	○ SPICY
○ THIN	○ CHUNKY

CHEESE TO SAUCE RATIO (CSR)

CHEESE	☐☐☐☐☐☐
SAUCE	☐☐☐☐☐☐

FRESHNESS

○1 ○2 ○3 ○4 ○5

CRUST SIZE

○ THIN
○ MEDIUM
○ LARGE

CRUST

○ BUTTERY	○ CRISPY
○ SPONGY	○ BUBBLY
○ CHEWY	○ OTHER

CRUST

○1 ○2 ○3 ○4 ○5

STYLE	○ NY ○ CHICAGO ○ OTHER

COMMENTS

MY RATING	○1 ○2 ○3 ○4 ○5 ○6 ○7 ○8 ○9 ○10	EAT AGAIN?	○ YES ○ NO

Pizza Log

DATE	
PIZZERIA	
NEIGHBORHOOD	

TOPPINGS

○ CHEESE	○ MUSHROOMS	○ ONIONS
○ PINEAPPLE	○ BACON	○ TUNA
○ GREEN PEPPER	○ SAUSAGE	○ BLACK OLIVES
○ OTHER		

CHEESE

○ GREASY	○ STINGY
○ SMOKEY	○ STINKY
○ CREAMY	○ SALTY

SAUCE

○ SWEET	○ SAVORY
○ TANGY	○ SPICY
○ THIN	○ CHUNKY

CHEESE TO SAUCE RATIO (CSR)

CHEESE	☐ ☐ ☐ ☐ ☐ ☐ ☐
SAUCE	☐ ☐ ☐ ☐ ☐ ☐ ☐

FRESHNESS

○1 ○2 ○3 ○4 ○5

CRUST SIZE / CRUST

CRUST SIZE	CRUST	
○ THIN	○ BUTTERY	○ CRISPY
○ MEDIUM	○ SPONGY	○ BUBBLY
○ LARGE	○ CHEWY	○ OTHER

CRUST

○1 ○2 ○3 ○4 ○5

STYLE	○ NY ○ CHICAGO ○ OTHER

COMMENTS

MY RATING	○1 ○2 ○3 ○4 ○5 ○6 ○7 ○8 ○9 ○10	EAT AGAIN?	○ YES ○ NO

Pizza Log

DATE	
PIZZERIA	
NEIGHBORHOOD	

TOPPINGS

○ CHEESE	○ MUSHROOMS	○ ONIONS
○ PINEAPPLE	○ BACON	○ TUNA
○ GREEN PEPPER	○ SAUSAGE	○ BLACK OLIVES

○ OTHER

CHEESE

○ GREASY	○ STINGY
○ SMOKEY	○ STINKY
○ CREAMY	○ SALTY

SAUCE

○ SWEET	○ SAVORY
○ TANGY	○ SPICY
○ THIN	○ CHUNKY

CHEESE TO SAUCE RATIO (CSR)

CHEESE	☐ ☐ ☐ ☐ ☐ ☐
SAUCE	☐ ☐ ☐ ☐ ☐ ☐

FRESHNESS

○1 ○2 ○3 ○4 ○5

CRUST SIZE / CRUST

CRUST SIZE	CRUST	
○ THIN	○ BUTTERY	○ CRISPY
○ MEDIUM	○ SPONGY	○ BUBBLY
○ LARGE	○ CHEWY	○ OTHER

CRUST

○1 ○2 ○3 ○4 ○5

STYLE	○ NY ○ CHICAGO ○ OTHER

COMMENTS

MY RATING	○1 ○2 ○3 ○4 ○5 ○6 ○7 ○8 ○9 ○10	EAT AGAIN?	○ YES ○ NO

Pizza Log

DATE	
PIZZERIA	
NEIGHBORHOOD	

TOPPINGS

○ CHEESE	○ MUSHROOMS	○ ONIONS
○ PINEAPPLE	○ BACON	○ TUNA
○ GREEN PEPPER	○ SAUSAGE	○ BLACK OLIVES
○ OTHER		

CHEESE

○ GREASY	○ STINGY
○ SMOKEY	○ STINKY
○ CREAMY	○ SALTY

SAUCE

○ SWEET	○ SAVORY
○ TANGY	○ SPICY
○ THIN	○ CHUNKY

CHEESE TO SAUCE RATIO (CSR)

CHEESE	☐ ☐ ☐ ☐ ☐ ☐
SAUCE	☐ ☐ ☐ ☐ ☐ ☐

FRESHNESS

○1 ○2 ○3 ○4 ○5

CRUST SIZE / CRUST

CRUST SIZE	CRUST	
○ THIN	○ BUTTERY	○ CRISPY
○ MEDIUM	○ SPONGY	○ BUBBLY
○ LARGE	○ CHEWY	○ OTHER

CRUST

○1 ○2 ○3 ○4 ○5

STYLE	○ NY ○ CHICAGO ○ OTHER

COMMENTS

MY RATING	○1 ○2 ○3 ○4 ○5 ○6 ○7 ○8 ○9 ○10	EAT AGAIN?	○ YES ○ NO

Pizza Log

DATE	
PIZZERIA	
NEIGHBORHOOD	

TOPPINGS

○ CHEESE	○ MUSHROOMS	○ ONIONS
○ PINEAPPLE	○ BACON	○ TUNA
○ GREEN PEPPER	○ SAUSAGE	○ BLACK OLIVES
○ OTHER		

CHEESE

○ GREASY	○ STINGY
○ SMOKEY	○ STINKY
○ CREAMY	○ SALTY

SAUCE

○ SWEET	○ SAVORY
○ TANGY	○ SPICY
○ THIN	○ CHUNKY

CHEESE TO SAUCE RATIO (CSR)

CHEESE	☐ ☐ ☐ ☐ ☐ ☐
SAUCE	☐ ☐ ☐ ☐ ☐ ☐

FRESHNESS

○1 ○2 ○3 ○4 ○5

CRUST SIZE

○ THIN	
○ MEDIUM	
○ LARGE	

CRUST

○ BUTTERY	○ CRISPY
○ SPONGY	○ BUBBLY
○ CHEWY	○ OTHER

CRUST

○1 ○2 ○3 ○4 ○5

STYLE	○ NY ○ CHICAGO ○ OTHER

COMMENTS

MY RATING	○1 ○2 ○3 ○4 ○5 ○6 ○7 ○8 ○9 ○10	EAT AGAIN?	○ YES ○ NO

www.ingramcontent.com/pod-product-compliance
Lightning Source LLC
Chambersburg PA
CBHW081232080526
44587CB00022B/3909